Upbility Publications LTD | 81–83 Grivas Digenis Avenue, Nicosia, 1090 Cyprus

E-mail: info@upbility.eu
www.upbility.net

SKU: EN-EB1123

Author: Aliki Kassotaki – Speech-Language Pathologist MSc, BSc

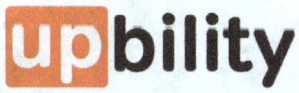

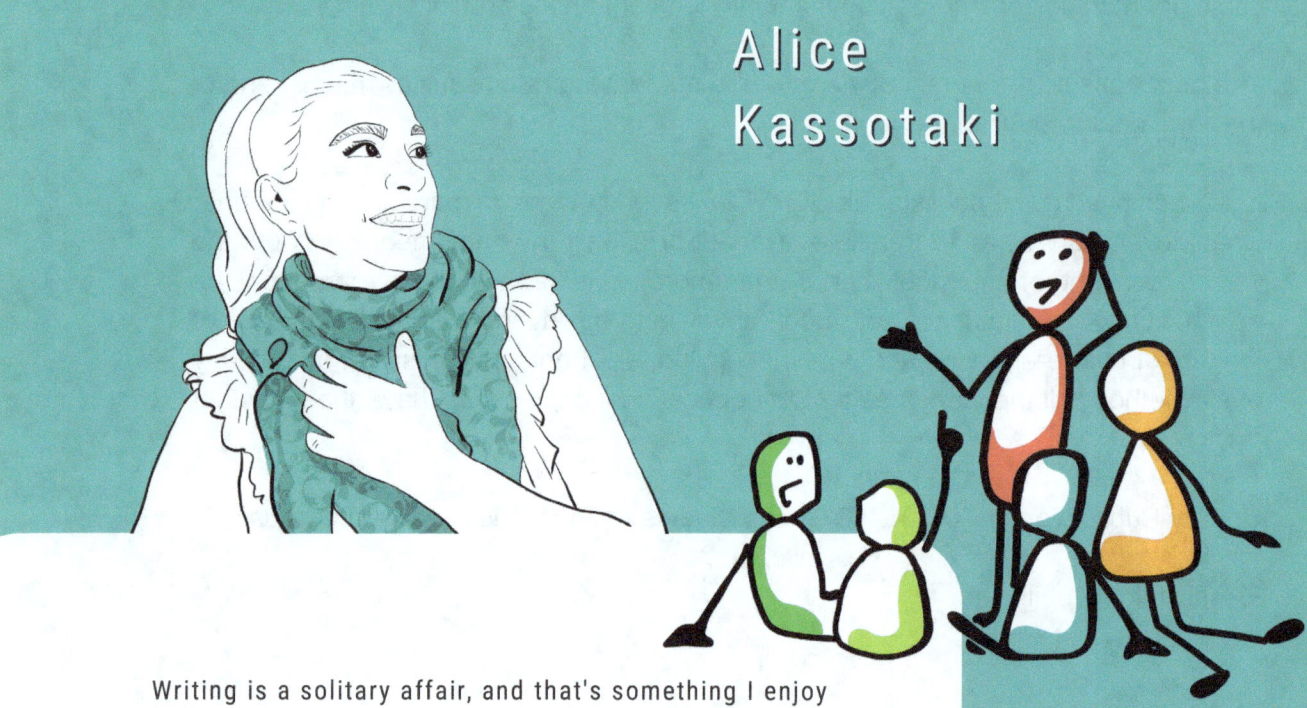

Alice Kassotaki

Writing is a solitary affair, and that's something I enjoy most of the time. Of course, I equally enjoy the company of my young and older students. I started working as a speech therapist in 2000. Thirteen years later, I wrote the first remedial manual. I wanted to share the knowledge and personal experience I have gained over the years. I have not stopped writing since then, and at the same time, I continue to practice my profession. One complements the other.

The children show me the way, and I join them in easy and challenging paths.

With empathy, humility, knowledge, and respect, I continue with my motto:
'Young children, fresh with uncluttered minds, the world before them - to what treasures will you lead them?'
Gladys M. Hunt

CONTENTS

Part A: Reading is the key to knowledge

1 Understanding stuttering

2 Causes of stuttering

3 Symptoms of stuttering

4 Diagnosis and evaluation of stuttering

5

Therapy For Stuttering

6

Living with stuttering

7

Myths and misconceptions about stuttering

Part B: From the books... to adventure

8

20 short stories

Introduction

Stuttering is a speech disorder that affects millions of people around the world. It's a condition that can significantly impact a person's life, affecting their self-esteem, social interactions, and ability to communicate effectively.

In the first part of this book, we delve into the topic of stuttering, exploring the causes, symptoms, diagnosis, and treatment options. We also discuss the various myths and misconceptions surrounding stuttering and how we can promote understanding and acceptance.

Children who stutter face unique challenges, including difficulty expressing themselves, interacting with others, and building self-confidence. As parents, carers, educators, and members of society, it's essential to understand the experiences of children who stutter and learn how to support them.

The second part presents 20 short stories describing social situations involving children and adolescents who stutter. We examine these stories from different perspectives, putting ourselves in the place of the stuttering child, the person interacting with the child, and the bystanders observing the situation. Each scenario is accompanied by an in-depth exploration of the thoughts, feelings, and possible actions of all parties involved.

The stories presented here are based on real experiences and aim to promote empathy, understanding, and awareness.

This book offers valuable insights to parents, teachers, and those who want to support a stuttering child through a comprehensive look into the complex social dynamics surrounding stuttering.

Whether you're a parent, a speech therapist, an educator, or someone who wants to learn more about stuttering, it's an essential resource for understanding and supporting children who stutter.

Part A

Reading is the key
to knowledge

1 Understanding stuttering

What is stuttering?

Stuttering is a speech disorder that affects the fluency and rhythm of speech. It's characterized by disruptions or pauses in the normal flow of speech, such as repetitions of sounds, syllables, words, prolongations, or blocks. Stuttering may also include physical expressions such as facial twitching or body movements in an attempt to produce speech. It's a neurological and developmental condition that usually occurs during childhood and may persist throughout adulthood. Stuttering can have significant social, emotional, and educational impacts on individuals. Still, with appropriate therapy, many people who stutter can significantly improve their speech fluency.

Effects and impact

Stuttering can significantly impact people who stutter both in terms of their communication skills and emotional well-being. Some of the effects of stuttering are:

Difficulties in communicating: Stuttering can make it difficult for individuals to communicate effectively, affecting their social, academic, or professional interactions.

© Upbility Publications

Negative emotions: Many people who stutter experience negative emotions related to their speech, such as anxiety, frustration, shame, or embarrassment.

Avoidance behaviors: Because of their negative emotions and fear of stuttering, some people who stutter may avoid speaking.

Self-esteem issues: Experiencing stuttering can negatively affect a person's self-esteem and self-confidence, especially if they face ridicule or negative reactions from others.

Social withdrawal: The negative effects of stuttering can lead some people to withdraw from social situations, resulting in loneliness and isolation.

What is developmental stuttering?

Developmental stuttering is a speech disorder that usually starts in childhood, between 2 and 4 years of age. It may include disorders in fluency, such as repetitions of sounds or words, prolongations of sounds, and blocking or hesitation before producing a sound or word.

Some children may overcome stuttering, while others may need treatment to improve their fluency.

Speech therapy is the most common form of treatment for developmental stuttering. It can help children learn strategies to reduce stuttering and improve their communication skills. In addition, support from parents, teachers, and peers can also help manage stuttering and boost a child's self-esteem and self-confidence.

What is neurogenic stuttering?

Neurogenic stuttering can occur due to neurological factors such as damage or injury to the brain or nervous system. It can result from various conditions, such as stroke, traumatic brain injury, Parkinson's disease, multiple sclerosis, and other neurological disorders.

Unlike developmental stuttering, which typically begins in childhood, neurogenic stuttering often occurs later in life, after neurological damage or injury. It's characterized by irregular and disrupted speech patterns, including repetitions, prolongations, and blocking.

Treatment of neurogenic stuttering may vary depending on the underlying cause and severity of the stuttering. Speech therapy may be helpful in some cases, as well as medication or other interventions to address the underlying neurological condition. In some cases, stuttering may be permanent, and the focus may shift to improving communication strategies and adapting to the condition.

What is psychogenic stuttering?

Psychogenic stuttering can be caused by psychological or emotional factors rather than neurological or developmental factors. It's often called "conversion disorder" because it involves converting emotional distress into physical symptoms such as stuttering.

It can occur as a response to a traumatic or stressful event such as abuse, a significant life change, or a traumatic experience. Psychogenic stuttering may also be a symptom of underlying mental health conditions such as anxiety, depression, or post-traumatic stress disorder.

Unlike developmental stuttering, psychogenic stuttering can have a sudden onset, and stuttering can come and go depending on the person's emotional state. Treatment for psychogenic stuttering may include addressing the underlying psychological or emotional factors through therapy or counseling and speech therapy to address the physical symptoms. In some cases, stuttering may get better on its own once the underlying emotional issues are addressed.

Causes of stuttering

2

Causes and factors that contribute to the occurrence and development of stuttering

The causes of stuttering are not fully understood. Still, research suggests that it may result from a combination of genetic, neurological, and environmental factors.

Genetics:

Stuttering tends to run in families, suggesting that there may be a genetic component to its development. Studies have identified several genes that may be associated with it.

Neurological factors:

Differences in brain structure and function may also lead to stuttering. Studies have found differences in the neural processing of language and speech in people who stutter.

Environmental factors:

Environmental factors, such as parenting behavior, stress, and trauma, can also lead to stuttering. Children who experience high levels of stress or trauma may be more likely to develop the condition.

Developmental factors:

Stuttering often occurs in childhood, when language and speech development move rapidly. Children with delays or difficulties in language development may be more likely to start stuttering.

Emotional factors:

Stress, low self-confidence, and other emotional factors can make stuttering worse or more challenging. These may be the cause of stuttering or result from it.

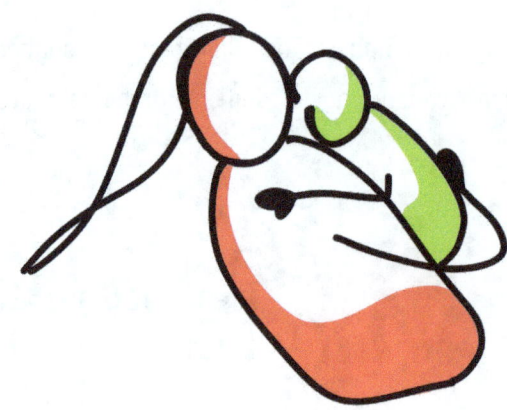

It's important to note that stuttering is a complex disorder, and the causes and factors leading to it may vary from person to person.

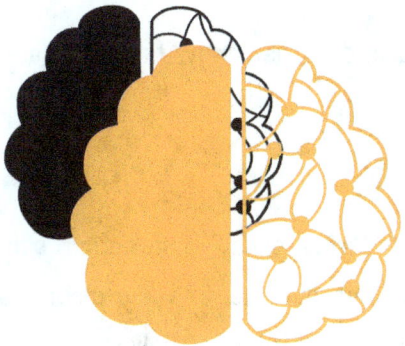

Structure and function of the brain

The structure and function of the brain play a significant role in the occurrence and development of stuttering.

Brain structure: Studies have found differences in the brain structure and function of people who stutter and those who don't. For example, they have shown differences in the size and connectivity of specific brain areas involved in language processing and speech production.

Brain function: Studies have also found differences in the neural processing of language and speech in people who stutter. For example, some studies have shown that stuttering may cause difficulty coordinating the movements involved in speech production.

Although the exact mechanisms underlying stuttering are not fully understood, research suggests that genetics, brain structure, and brain function may interact in complicated ways and contribute to the disorder. Eventually, understanding these factors may help develop more effective treatments for stuttering.

Association between stuttering and other communication disorders

Stuttering is a speech disorder that may be associated or coexist with other communication disorders.

Language disorders:

Children who stutter may also experience language development difficulties, such as vocabulary or phonology delays. This may be related to underlying brain function or structure differences that lead to stuttering and language disorders.

Voice disorders:

Stuttering can also be associated with voice disorders such as vocal nodules or polyps. These disorders can lead to changes in voice quality and may worsen the symptoms of stuttering.

Social communication disorder:

A social communication disorder is characterized by problems in social interaction and communication, including difficulties in understanding and using non-verbal language. Children who stutter may also experience difficulties in social communication, leading to feelings of isolation and social anxiety.

Autism spectrum disorder:

Autism spectrum disorder is characterized by difficulties in social interaction, communication, and repetitive behaviors. Although stuttering is not a typical symptom of autism, some children with autism may also experience stuttering.

Selective mutism:

Selective mutism is characterized by an inability to speak in specific social situations, despite being able to speak in other cases. Some children who stutter may also have selective mutism, which makes communicating effectively in social situations difficult.

It is important to note that while these disorders may coexist with stuttering, not all children who stutter have them.

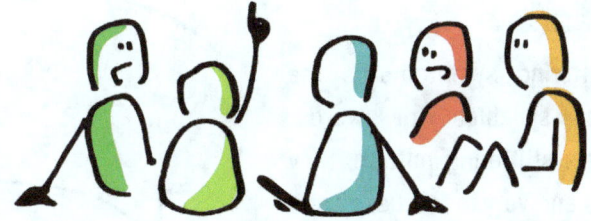

Symptoms of
3 stuttering

Stuttering is a speech disorder characterized by disruptions in fluency and rhythm of speech. Some common symptoms are:

REPETITIONS

One of the main stuttering symptoms is the repetition of sounds, syllables, or words. Depending on someone's stuttering pattern, they can take different forms and vary in frequency and duration.

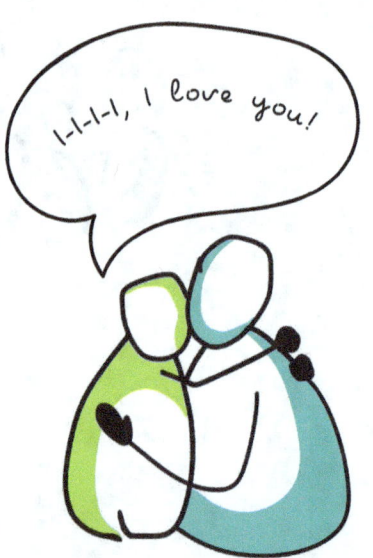

I-I-I-I, I love you!

Repetition of sounds: It occurs when someone repeats the initial sound of a word, such as "b-b-b-bye." Sound repetitions may also occur in the middle or end of words.

Repetition of syllables: It occurs when someone repeats a syllable of a word, such as "ki-ki-ki-kitchen."

Repetition of words: It occurs when someone repeats a whole word, such as "sit-sit-sit down."

The repetitions may be short or prolonged and may be accompanied by tension in the facial or body muscles. Some people may try to avoid repetitions by substituting words or using complementary words such as "um" or "ah" to fill pauses in their speech.

Repetitions can significantly impact a person's communication skills and lead to frustration and embarrassment. Speech therapy can help reduce the frequency and severity of repetitions and improve overall communication skills.

PROLONGATIONS

Another common symptom of stuttering is prolongation, which occurs when a person prolongs or extends the duration of a sound during speech.

Sound prolongations: They occur when someone prolongs the sound of a word, such as "ppppput."

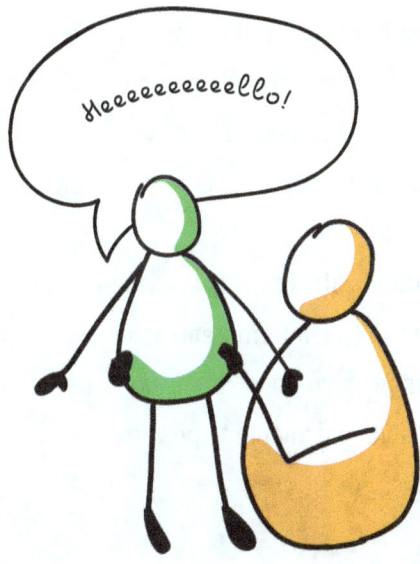

Prolongations are often accompanied by visible tension in the facial or body muscles, and the person may struggle to release the sound or syllable to move on to the next word.

As with repetitions, prolongations can lead to frustration, anxiety, and embarrassment, negatively affecting communication skills and social Interactions. Speech therapy can be beneficial in reducing the frequency and severity of prolongations and teaching the individual to use techniques to improve fluency and overall communication skills.

It is important to note that prolongations and repetitions may occur together or separately and that each person's stuttering pattern is unique. The severity and frequency of stuttering can also vary over time and may be affected by factors such as stress, fatigue, and excitement.

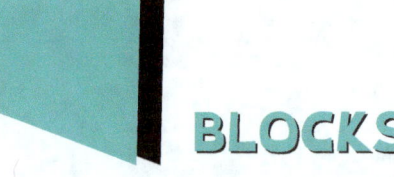

BLOCKS

Blocks are another common symptom of stuttering, which occurs when someone experiences a sudden pause in their speech. Blocks can take various forms, such as:

Silent block: It occurs when someone tries to speak, but no sound comes out. They may seem to struggle to release the sound or word and feel tension in their face or body muscles.

Auditory block: It occurs when someone produces a partial or intermittent sound such as "k...". The person may seem stuck on a particular sound or syllable and unable to progress in their speech.

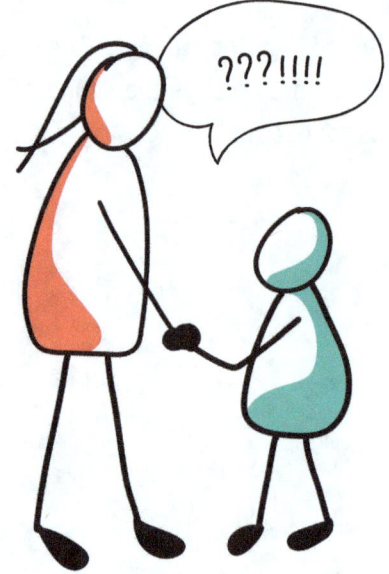

Repeated block: It occurs when someone experiences blocks, repetitions, or prolongations within a word or phrase, such as "b-b-b-bunny."

Blocks can be particularly frustrating and embarrassing for people who stutter, as they can disrupt the flow of conversation and make it challenging to communicate effectively. They can also lead to avoiding certain words or situations, limiting the person's social and professional opportunities.

Speech therapy can help teach people who stutter strategies to manage and reduce the severity of blocks, such as gentle speech initiation, slow and controlled breathing, and relaxation techniques. Such techniques can help improve a stutterer's fluency and confidence.

SECONDARY BEHAVIORS

Tension or struggling of the facial or body muscles during speech is a common stuttering feature. When a person experiences stuttering, they may exhibit secondary behaviors. These physical or verbal responses occur in response to the tension or struggle during stuttering. Some examples of secondary behaviors are:

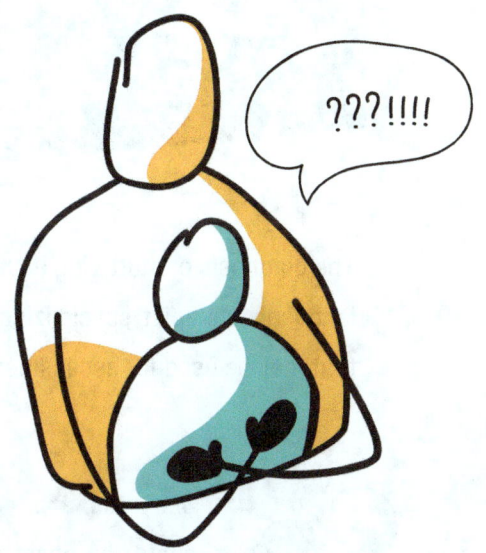

Facial tension: Someone who stutters may tighten their facial muscles when speaking, doing things like clenching their jaw, squinting their eyes, or raising their eyebrows.

Body tension: Someone who stutters may show tension in their body when speaking, doing things like clenching their fists, stretching their shoulders or neck, or shaking their body.

Avoidance behaviors: Someone who stutters may avoid speaking in certain situations or avoid certain words or sounds that cause their stuttering. For example, they may avoid talking on the phone or using the "s" phoneme.

Interjections or filler words: ASomeone who stutters may use filler words or interjections such as "um" or "ah" to fill pauses in their speech or avoid stuttering on a particular word or sound.

These secondary behaviors can become habits that are difficult to break and can exacerbate the negative effects of stuttering. They can also cause additional anxiety and stress to the stutterer.

It's important to note that everyone's experience with stuttering is unique, and symptoms can vary in frequency and severity over time. If you or someone you know have any symptoms, it's recommended that you see a speech and language therapist for evaluation and treatment.

Diagnosis and evaluation of stuttering

4

The diagnosis of stuttering usually involves a comprehensive evaluation by a speech and language therapist specializing in treating fluency disorders. Here are some methods that may be used for assessment:

 **Background information:** The therapist may ask the person or family about the onset of stuttering, family history of stuttering, and any other relevant information.

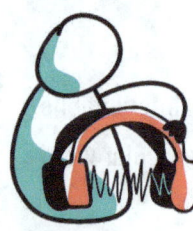 **Speech sample analysis:** The therapist may analyze speech samples to determine the frequency and severity of stuttering. The speech sample may be taken during a conversation (spontaneous speech) or reading.

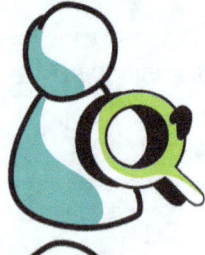 **Observation:** The therapist may observe the person's speech during various activities.

 **Standardized tests:** The therapist may use standardized tests to assess the person's phonological and language skills, as well as their cognitive and socio-emotional function.

Self-reference measures: The therapist may use self-report measures to assess the individual's perception of their stuttering.

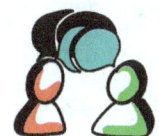

Functional assessment: The therapist may assess the impact of the stuttering on the individual's daily life in instances like social interactions, academic performance, and emotional well-being.

Non-Standardized tests: Depending on the individual's needs, the therapist may conduct additional informal testing for a more comprehensive evaluation.

Overall, the assessment process is customized to the individual's unique needs and may include a combination of these methods. The goal of the evaluation is to provide an accurate diagnosis and create an individualized treatment plan that meets the specific needs and objectives of the individual.

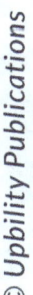

Evaluation tools and approaches

There are various assessment tools and approaches used by speech and language therapists to evaluate stuttering, such as:

Stuttering Severity Instrument (SSI): SSI is a widely used tool to measure the frequency, duration, and physical characteristics of stuttering. It's suitable for people of all ages and provides a numerical score indicating stuttering severity.

Overall assessment of the speaker's experience of stuttering (OASES): OASES is a self-report measure that assesses the impact of stuttering on the person's daily life. It covers four domains: communication, reactions to stuttering, quality of life, and environment.

Fluency shaping therapy: This approach focuses on teaching people techniques to control their stuttering, such as speaking at a slower pace or using soft word onset. The effectiveness of this approach can be evaluated through measures such as speech rate, fluency rate, and stuttering severity.

Stuttering modification therapy: This approach aims to help individuals modify their stuttering behaviors by reducing the intensity or avoiding word repetition. The effectiveness of this approach can be evaluated through measures such as the number of disfluencies and speech rate.

Cognitive behavioral therapy (CBT): CBT aims to address the negative emotions and thoughts associated with stuttering. Assessing the effectiveness of CBT may include measures such as self-report measures of anxiety and depression, as well as changes in attitudes and communication behaviors.

Overall, assessment tools and approaches to stuttering are customized to the unique needs and objectives of the individual. The choice of assessment tools and methods depends on factors such as someone's age, the severity of their stuttering, and the treatment goals.

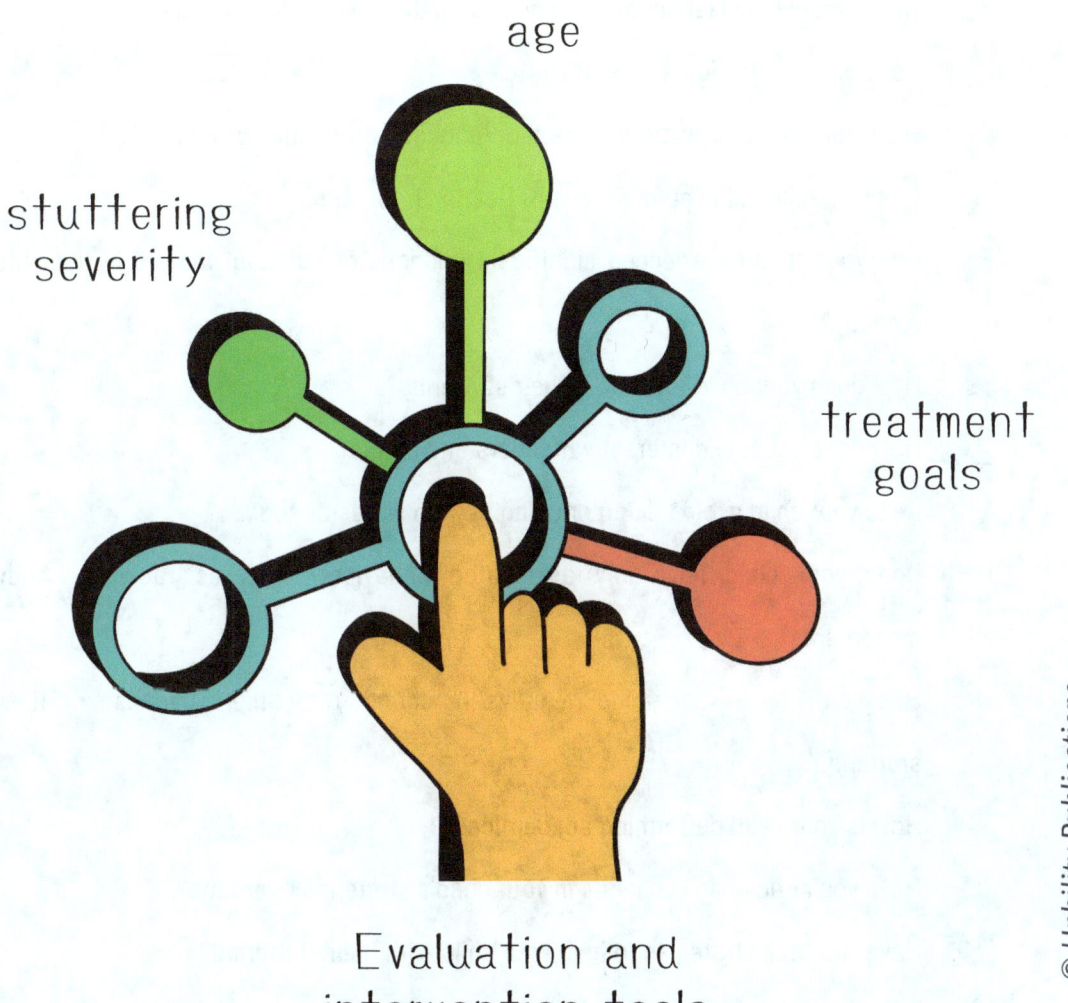

age

stuttering
severity

treatment
goals

Evaluation and
intervention tools

Questionnaire for parents

The following are questions a speech and language therapist may ask the parents of a child who stutters.

1 When did you first notice your child's stuttering?

2 Does your child stutter more during certain activities or situations?

3 Does your child seem to be aware of their stuttering?

4 Has a speech and language therapist evaluated your child in the past?

5 Does anyone else in the family stutter?

6 Have you noticed any other speech or language difficulties in your child?

7 Has your child had ear infections or hearing problems?

8 Has your child experienced significant changes or stressful factors in their life recently?

9 How does your child feel about their stuttering?

10 How does your child interact with peers and adults?

11 Does your child avoid talking or using certain words or sounds?

12 Does your child have any associated behaviors, such as facial or body movements?

13 Has your child experienced negative reactions from others because of their stuttering?

14 How is your child performing academically?

15 Have you noticed any changes in your child's stuttering over time?

16 Have you tried strategies to help your child with their stuttering?

17 What are your concerns about your child's stuttering?

18 How does your child's stuttering affect their daily life?

19 Are there other factors that may contribute to your child's stuttering, such as stress or a neurological condition?

20 What are your goals for improving your child's communication skills?

Questionnaire for children/ adolescents

The following are questions a speech and language therapist may ask a school-age child or teenager who stutters.

1. Can you tell me when you first noticed that you stutter?

2. How does stuttering make you feel?

3. Are there instances when you stutter more than usual? What are they?

4. Do you know anyone else who stutters?

5. Do you feel people treat you differently because of your stuttering?

6. Do you avoid certain words or situations because you are afraid of stuttering?

7. Can you recall an instance you felt particularly good about your speech?

8. Can you recall an instance when you felt particularly bad about your speech?

9. What do you think causes your stuttering?

10. Do you have any questions or concerns about your speech or stuttering?

11. How do you feel when you speak in front of your class?

12. How do you feel when you talk on the phone?

13. Are there any words (or sounds) that you have more difficulty saying than others?

14. How does your stuttering affect your ability to participate in activities you enjoy?

15. Do you ever feel anxious or nervous when you talk?

16. Have you ever tried any techniques to help you with your stuttering?

17. Do you feel your stuttering is improving, worsening, or staying the same?

18. How does your stuttering affect your relationships with family and friends?

19. What are your goals for improving your speech and communication?

20. Is there anything else you want me to know about your stuttering?

Therapy For Stuttering

5

Therapeutic approach

Speech therapy

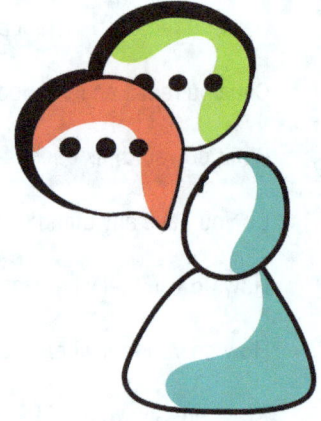

This approach focuses on improving a person's fluency through various techniques such as:

Stuttering modification therapy: This approach helps individuals identify and modify their stuttering behaviors by reducing volume or avoiding word repetition.

Fluency modulation therapy: This approach teaches individuals techniques to control their stuttering, like speaking at a slower pace or using soft onset phonation.

Integrated approach: This approach combines stuttering modification and fluency modulation techniques to help individuals achieve more comfortable speech.

Psychotherapy

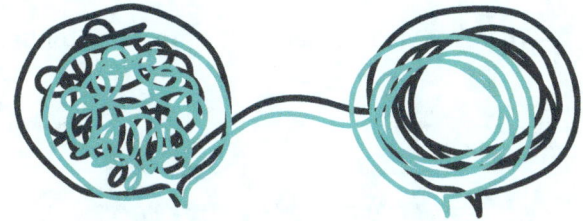

This approach addresses the emotional and psychological aspects of stuttering, such as anxiety, self-esteem, and communication attitudes. Psychotherapy may include:

Cognitive-behavioral therapy (CBT): This approach helps individuals change negative thinking patterns and behaviors that may contribute to their stuttering, such as avoiding talking situations.

Acceptance and Commitment Therapy (ACT): This approach helps individuals develop acceptance and mindfulness skills to manage the negative thinking and feelings associated with their stuttering.

Supportive therapy: This approach provides a safe and supportive place for individuals to discuss their experiences with stuttering and develop coping strategies.

Both speech therapy and psychotherapy can be effective in treating stuttering. Choosing the proper treatment approach depends on the individual's unique needs and goals, the severity of their stuttering, and its impact on their daily life. A combined approach, including speech therapy and psychotherapy, may also benefit some individuals.

© Upbility Publications

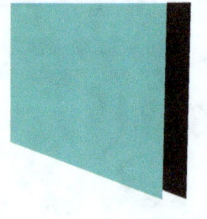

Therapeutic programs

There are various therapeutic programs for treating stuttering, such as:

Lidcombe Program:

The Lidcombe program is a behavioral treatment for preschool children who stutter. Parents are encouraged to provide feedback to their children about their stuttering using positive and negative reinforcement. The program is based on functional scaling, where positive reinforcement increases desirable behaviors (e.g., fluency), and negative reinforcement decreases undesirable behaviors (e.g., stuttering).

Palin Parent-Child Interaction Therapy:

Palin Parent-Child Interaction Therapy is a therapeutic program for children who stutter. It's based on the Lidcombe program and involves a structured approach to parent-child conversations that encourage smooth speech.

FluencyBank:

FluencyBank is a computer-based program that provides feedback to people who stutter. The program uses visual and auditory feedback to help individuals achieve more fluent speech.

The Camperdown Program:

The Camperdown program is a treatment for adults who stutter. It involves speech restructuring, which teaches individuals to speak more slowly and with controlled breathing. The program also incorporates cognitive-behavioral therapy techniques to address the anxiety and negative thinking associated with stuttering.

Stuttering Modification Therapy:

Stuttering modification therapy is a therapeutic approach that focuses on modifying stuttering behaviors, such as reducing the intensity or avoiding repetitive words. Therapy helps individuals develop coping strategies to manage their stuttering and improve their communication skills.

These therapeutic programs vary in their approaches and techniques, and the choice of the program depends on the individual's unique needs and goals. A speech-language pathologist can assist someone in determining which program is most appropriate for them based on age, condition severity, family profile, and treatment goals.

The role of family and support systems in treating stuttering

Family and support systems can play an essential role in treating stuttering by helping individuals in several ways, such as:

Education and raising awareness: Family members and support systems can learn about stuttering and its impact on communication and daily life. This way, they will understand how the person experiences stuttering and how to support them.

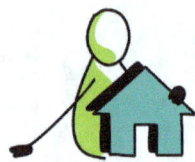

Home practice: Speech and language therapy can include exercises and strategies for home practice. Family members and support systems can reinforce these strategies and provide a supportive environment for the individual to practice communication skills.

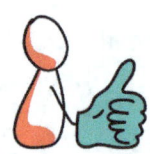

Positive reinforcement: Family members and support systems can provide positive feedback and support for the individual's communication efforts. That way, they can help boost their confidence and motivate them to continue practicing their skills.

Support groups: Family members and support systems can guide the individual to the available support groups and community resources. That way, they can provide them with a sense of community and reduce feelings of isolation associated with stuttering.

Overall, the involvement of family members and support systems can create a supportive environment for the individual to practice communication skills, reduce feelings of isolation and stigmatization, and improve their overall quality of life.

6 Living with stuttering

Challenges and opportunities:

Living with stuttering can be very challenging, but it can also provide opportunities for growth and self-awareness.

Challenges

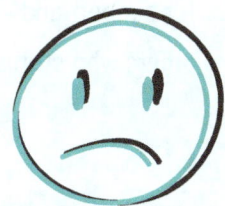

Communication difficulties: Stuttering can make communicating difficult, leading to frustration and anxiety. Fear of stuttering can also cause individuals to avoid certain social situations or conversations.

Negative reactions: Stuttering can lead to negative responses from others, such as teasing or bullying, which can significantly impact a person's self-esteem and self-confidence.

Educational challenges: Stuttering can also affect academic performance, as individuals may struggle with oral presentations or classroom discussions.

Social isolation: Stuttering can also lead to social isolation, as individuals may feel embarrassed or unconfident about their speech and avoid social situations.

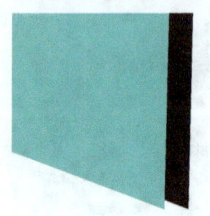

Opportunities

Building resilience and coping skills: Living with stuttering can help individuals develop resilience and coping skills as they learn to deal with the challenges associated with their disorder.

Personal development: Living with stuttering can lead to personal growth and self-awareness as individuals learn to accept and embrace their condition as part of their identity.

Defending and empowering: Living with stuttering can also provide opportunities for support and empowerment as individuals often need to protect themselves and others who stutter and promote awareness and acceptance.

Positive relationships: Living with stuttering can also lead to positive relationships as individuals learn to form supportive and accepting relationships with others who understand and accept their condition.

When educating a child or adolescent who stutters, it's vital to provide opportunities and support them to succeed academically and socially. This may include collaborating with the school to develop a plan to provide extra time for oral presentations or speech therapy services to improve their communication skills. It's also important to create a supportive environment at home and in the community to help the child or adolescent and make them feel accepted and respected. This can help them develop their self-esteem and confidence, improving their overall well-being and future success.

Tips and strategies for dealing with stuttering

Here are some tips and strategies for dealing with stuttering in children and adolescents:

 Slowing down: Encourage the child or adolescent to slow down, take their time, and use pauses to help reduce stuttering.

 Relaxation techniques: Teach the child or adolescent relaxation techniques, such as deep breathing or progressive muscle relaxation, to help reduce the tension and anxiety associated with stuttering.

 Easy onsets: Encourage the child or adolescent to use easy onset techniques such as starting a word gently and gradually increasing the volume to help reduce stuttering.

 Observing breathing: Teach the child or teen to monitor their breathing while speaking and take deep breaths before speaking to reduce tension and facilitate fluency.

 Practicing fluency techniques: Work with a speech and language therapist to develop and practice fluency-improving techniques, such as slow and controlled speech.

 Positive self-talk: Encourage the child or adolescent to use positive self-talk and affirmations, such as "I am a good communicator," to boost self-confidence and reduce negative thinking and feelings associated with stuttering.

 Supportive environment: Create a supportive environment at home and in the community that encourages open communication and acceptance of stuttering.

 Communication strategies: Encourage the child or adolescent to develop effective communication strategies, such as asking for time to collect their thoughts or using alternative forms of communicating, like writing or typing.

© Upbility Publications

Professional help: Seek a speech and language therapist to develop a personalized treatment plan and provide the child with ongoing support and guidance.

 Connect with support groups: Connect with support groups and organizations that provide resources and support to people who stutter and their families.

These tips and strategies can help children and adolescents who stutter develop effective communication skills, boost self-confidence and self-esteem, and reduce negative thinking and feelings associated with stuttering. It's also essential to work with a speech and language therapist and create a supportive environment to ensure the best possible outcomes for the child or adolescent.

Myths and misconceptions about stuttering

7

1. Stuttering is caused by anxiety or stress.

2. Stuttering is a sign of low intelligence.

3. People who stutter lack self-confidence or self-esteem.

4. Stuttering is caused by a lack of willpower or laziness.

5. Stuttering is a rare disorder.

6. Stuttering can be cured by simply slowing down or taking a deep breath.

7. Stuttering is caused by parents or family members talking too fast or badly.

8. People who stutter are not social.

9. All children recover from stuttering on their own.

10. Stuttering is a psychological disorder that can only be treated with therapy.

Small and big truths about stuttering

7

1 Stuttering is a neurological condition that affects speech fluency.

2 Stuttering is not caused by stress or nervousness, although these factors can make stuttering worse in some people.

3 People who stutter have normal intelligence and can be successful in all areas of life.

4 Stuttering does not indicate a lack of self-confidence or self-esteem.

5 Stuttering affects about 1% of the world's population, making it a relatively common condition.

6 Although there is no known cure for stuttering, there are effective treatment options that can help individuals manage their stuttering and improve their communication skills.

7 A lack of willpower or laziness does not cause stuttering, and individuals who stutter are not to blame for their condition.

8 People who stutter can be excellent at communicating and may have unique perspectives and skills as a result of their experiences with stuttering.

9 Early intervention and support for children who stutter can be crucial to help them develop healthy communication habits and manage their stuttering.

10 Stuttering is a complex condition that can occur differently in each individual, so it's important to approach a person's experience with empathy and understanding.

Part B

From the books...

to adventure

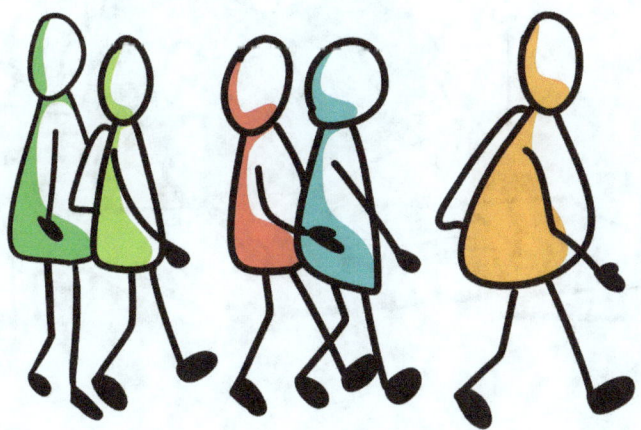

Reading aloud

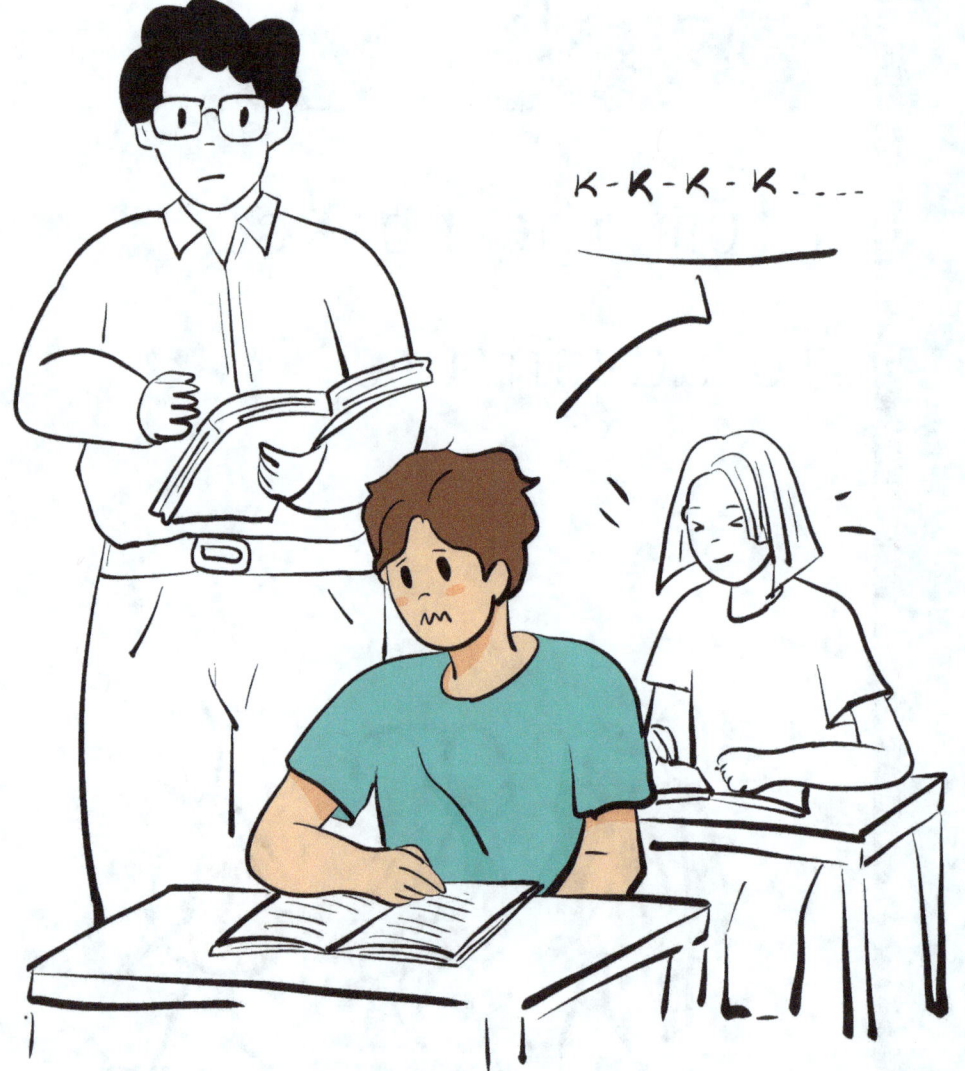

K-K-K-K....

Tom is asked to read aloud in class but he stutters, causing the other students to giggle and make fun of him.

Story analysis

From Tom's perspective

A. Thoughts and feelings:

Tom may feel...

- Embarrassed and humiliated when other students make fun of him.
- Anxious when reading aloud in front of others because of his stuttering.
- Disappointed that he cannot read smoothly and fluently like his classmates.
- Lonely and without the support of his classmates and teacher.

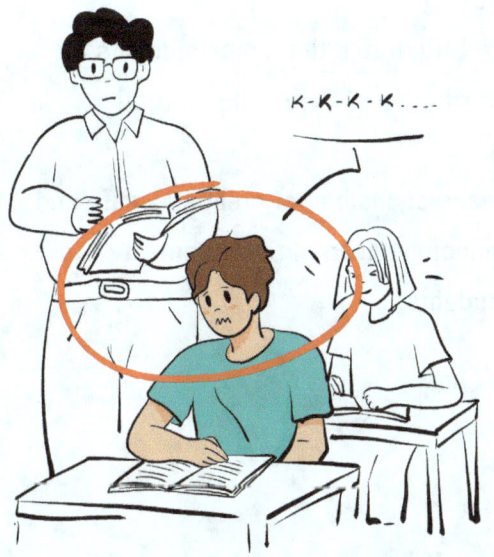

B. Possible actions:

- Tom may avoid reading aloud in class or refuse to attend school.
- Tom may develop low self-esteem and self-confidence.
- Tom may feel anger and resentment towards his classmates and teacher.
- Tom may seek help from a speech and language therapist or counselor to overcome his stuttering and improve his communication skills.

Story analysis

From the teacher's perspective

A. Thoughts and feelings:

The teacher may...

- Feel empathy for Tom and understand the challenges he faces due to his stuttering.
- Feel frustrated that some students are making fun of Tom and interrupting class.
- Feel responsible for creating a safe and welcoming learning environment for all students.

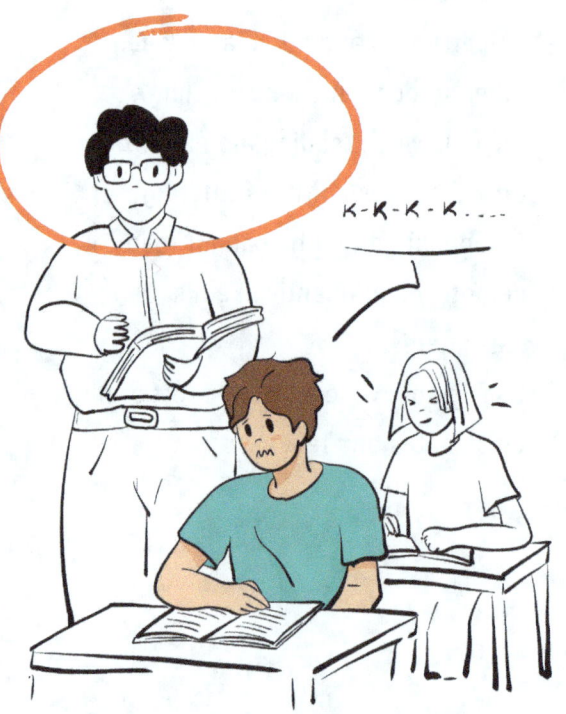

B. Possible actions:

The teacher may...

- Intervene when other students make fun of Tom and explain why this is hurtful and disrespectful.
- Offer support and encouragement to Tom and praise him for his efforts.
- Work with Tom's parents and a speech and language therapist to develop a plan to help him overcome his stuttering and improve his reading skills.
- Educate the class about stuttering and communication disorders to promote awareness and understanding.

Story analysis

From the perspective of bystanders

A. Thoughts and feelings:

- Some students may find Tom's stuttering amusing and enjoy making fun of him.
- Other students may be uncomfortable or embarrassed by the situation and not know how to react.
- Some students may feel sympathy for Tom and wish they could help him.

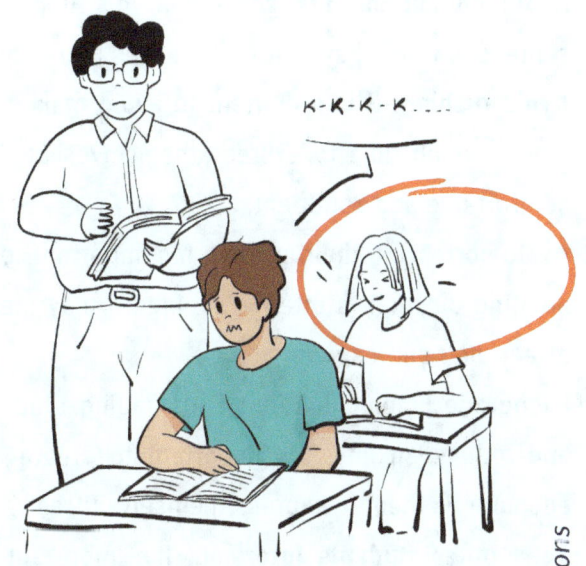

B. Possible actions:

- Some students may continue making fun of Tom and contributing to a hostile educational environment.
- Other students may speak out against bullying and support Tom.
- Some students may try to befriend Tom and help him feel included in the classroom.
- Some students may feel powerless and unable to help Tom or improve the situation.

Story analysis

Tips for effective communication:

Maintain eye contact: Maintaining eye contact with the person stuttering while speaking is a sign of respect and understanding. It also helps them feel comfortable and confident when expressing themselves.

Avoid completing his sentences: It's important to avoid completing the student's sentences when they stutter. It causes more anxiety for the student.

Avoid rushing: It is important to avoid making the student rush when speaking. Giving them enough time to express themselves at their own pace will make them feel more comfortable and confident.

Avoid correcting their speech: It's important to avoid correcting the student's speech or pointing out their stuttering. Doing so may make them feel embarrassed and may also affect their self-esteem.

Encourage communication: Encouraging students to speak can help build confidence and reduce anxiety. It's important to create a safe and supportive environment that encourages them to express themselves freely.

Keep other students informed: It's important to educate other students in the class about stuttering and how it affects people. Encourage them to be patient, understanding and avoid making fun of students who stutter.

Effective communication with people who stutter requires patience, understanding, and empathy. By following these tips, teachers can create a supportive learning environment that helps students who stutter feel comfortable and confident when communicating.

© Upbility Publications

Story analysis

Summary

It's important that all parties involved take specific actions. The child and parents can seek help from a speech and language therapist or health counselor to develop coping strategies for the child's stuttering and improve their communication skills. The teacher can provide support and encouragement to the child, intervene when other students are making fun of the child, and educate the class about stuttering and communication disorders. Other bystanders can support the child, speak out against bullying and try to include the child in social interactions in the classroom.

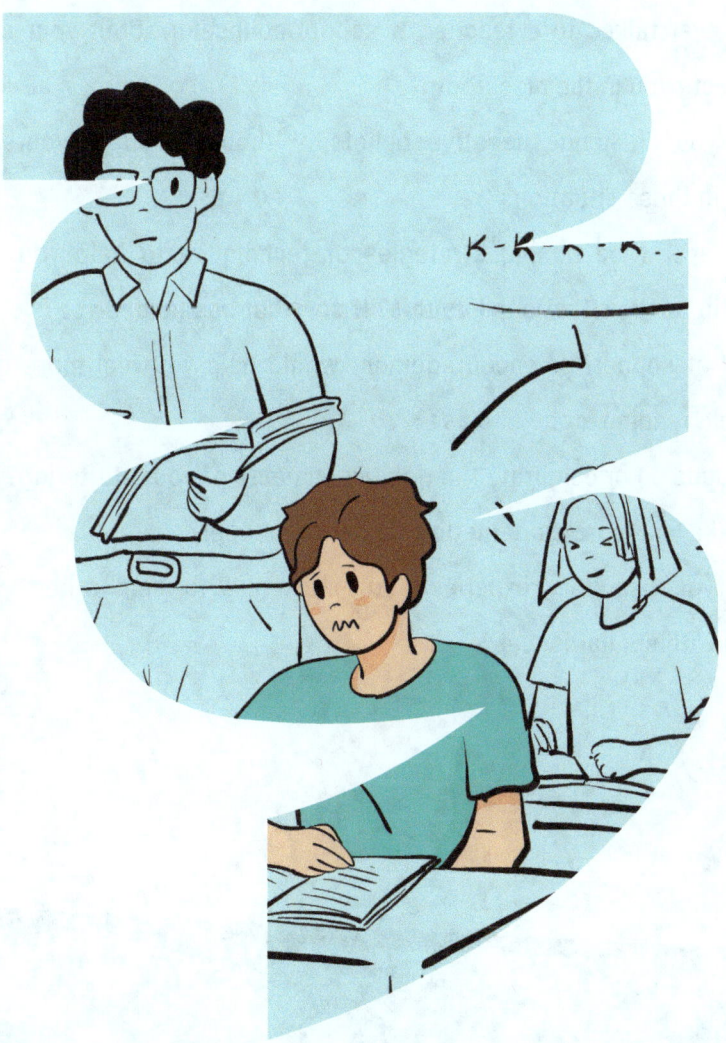

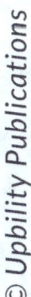

1

Story analysis

Questions...

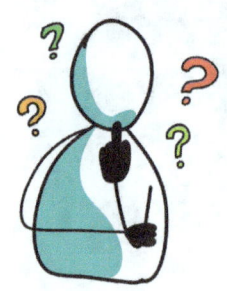

1. On a scale of 1 to 10 (1 = very little, 10 = very much), how much do you think Tom stutters?

2. How often do you struggle with stuttering in public situations, such as reading aloud in class?

3. What feelings or emotions do you experience when you stutter and others laugh or make fun of you?

4. How do you usually react to others teasing or laughing at you in these situations?

5. Do you feel that your stuttering defines who you are as a person? Why or why not?

6. Have you ever talked to a teacher or school counselor about your stuttering and how it affects you in the classroom?

7. How can you challenge negative beliefs or thoughts about yourself and your stuttering in these situations?

8. Have you ever tried coping strategies or techniques to help you manage your stuttering in public situations like this? If so, what has helped you?

9. What kind of support or encouragement would help you feel more confident and comfortable reading aloud in class?

10. Can you focus on or celebrate the positive aspects of your stuttering? For example, does it make you more empathetic or a better listener?

11. How can you use your experience of stuttering to help others who may be struggling with similar issues?

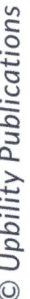

2 At the restaurant

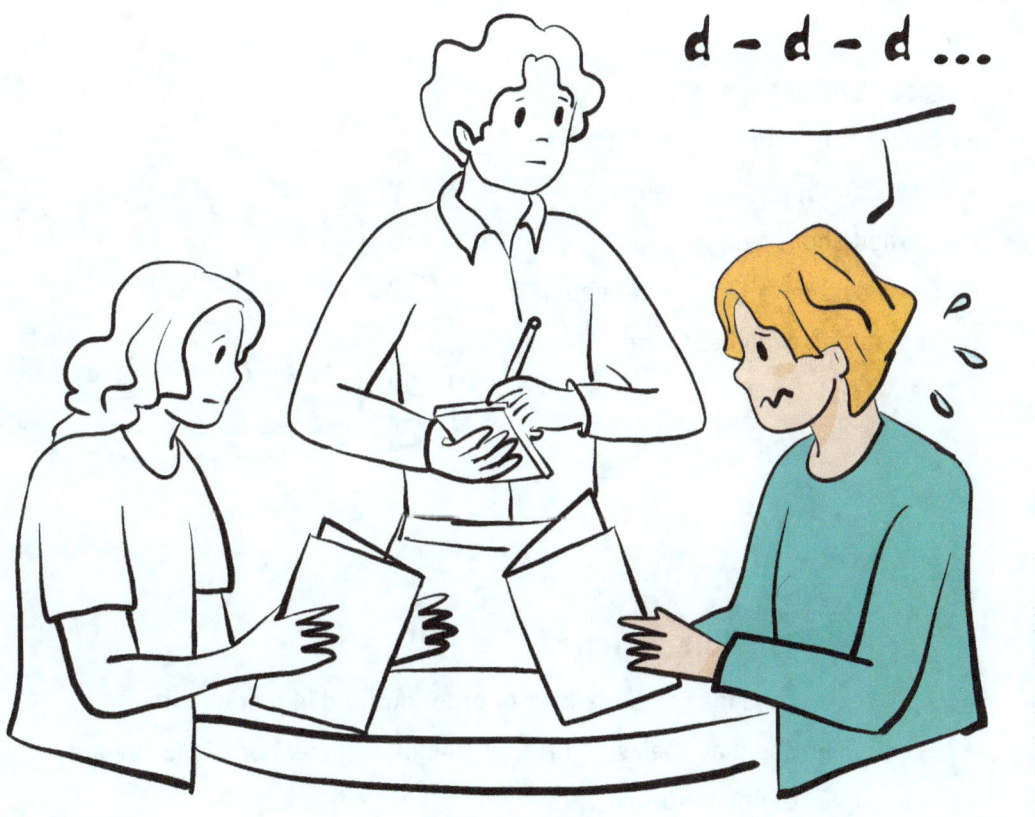

Lena visits a restaurant with her friend but has difficulty ordering food because she stutters, and the waiter cannot understand what she wants.

Story analysis

From Lena's perspective

A. Thoughts and feelings:

Lena may feel...

- Disappointed and embarrassed about her stuttering.
- Stressed because she is not being understood, further causing her anxiety and low confidence in her speech.
- Concerned about being judged or ridiculed by the waiter or other people in the restaurant, even her friend.

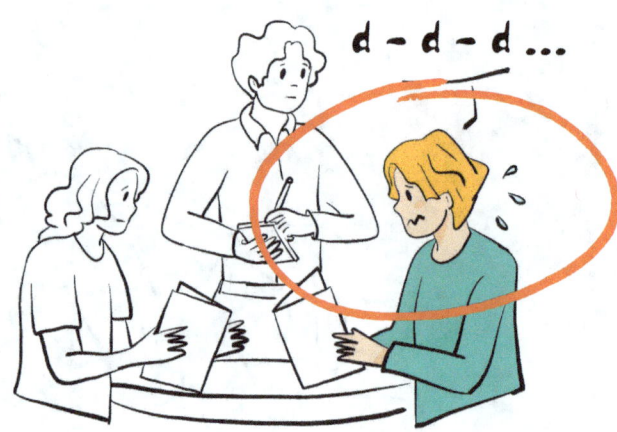

B. Possible actions:

- Lena may avoid talking or ordering food in restaurants.
- She may seek support from family members or friends aware of her stuttering.
- She may use alternative methods of communication, such as writing her order or pointing to pictures on the menu.

2 Story analysis

From the waiter's perspective

A. Thoughts and feelings:

The waiter may...

- Feel confused or frustrated by Lena's speech difficulties, especially if he is not familiar with stuttering.
- Worry about holding up the queue or making other customers wait.
- Want to provide good customer service but lack the knowledge to communicate effectively.

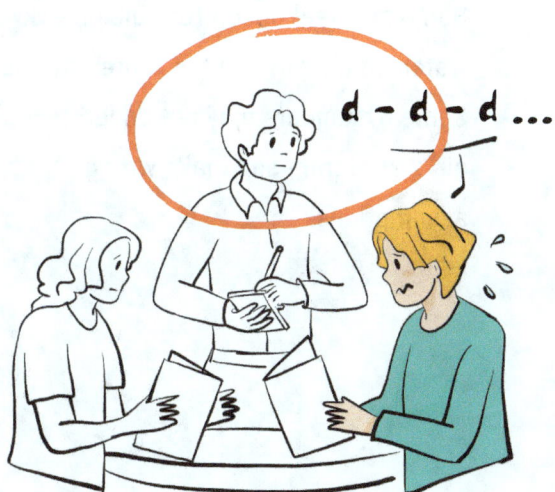

B. Possible actions:

The waiter may...

- Try to make Lena hurry or become impatient, worsening her anxiety and making it even more difficult for her to communicate.
- Seek guidance or training on how to communicate effectively with people who stutter.
- Try to use non-verbal cues or provide visual aids to help Lena understand menu options.
- Wait patiently for her to complete her sentence.

2 Story analysis

From the perspective of bystanders

A. Thoughts and feelings:

- Bystanders may feel sympathy for the girl and want to help.
- Some may feel uncomfortable or awkward watching the girl and the waiter interact.
- Some bystanders may not understand the girl's stuttering and make wrong assumptions.

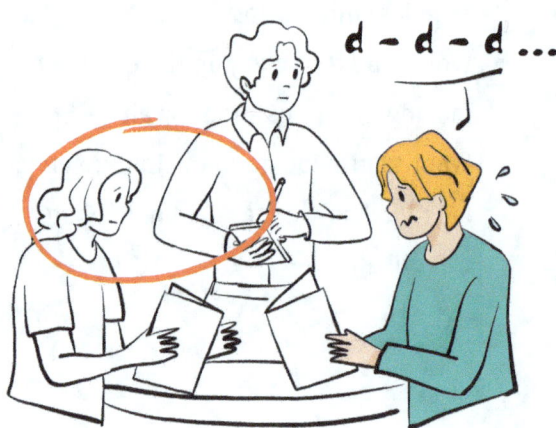

B. Possible actions:

- The bystanders may be patient and respectful to the girl and the waiter.
- They may offer to help the child communicate her order or provide support and encouragement.
- They may seek to be educated about stuttering and supporting people who stutter.

2 Story analysis

Tips for effective communication:

Be patient: Give Lena enough time to complete her sentences without interrupting or finishing them. This will make her feel more comfortable and less stressed.

Maintain eye contact: Show that you are actively listening and participating in the conversation by maintaining eye contact. This shows respect and encourages Lena to keep talking.

Avoid making assumptions: Avoid guessing what Lena is trying to say or making assumptions about her order. Instead, politely wait for her to express herself and clarify something if necessary.

Ask for clarification: If you are having trouble understanding Lena's order, ask her to repeat or clarify it. You can also suggest that she points to the item on the menu if that would be easier for her.

Offer alternatives: If Lena has difficulty verbally expressing her order, offer alternative methods of communication, such as writing it down or typing it on a smartphone.

Stay calm and positive: Maintain a friendly and supportive attitude throughout the interaction. This will create a more comfortable environment for Lena and help her relax.

Be sensitive and empathetic: Acknowledge Lena's stuttering without making her feel embarrassed or uncomfortable. Show empathy and understanding, which will help her feel more supported and less anxious.

Educate himself: Learn more about stuttering and its effects on communication. This will help you better understand the challenges Lena may be facing and allow you to support her better.

Story analysis

Summary

In conclusion, it's important to be patient and understanding when communicating with someone who stutters. Always maintain eye contact and actively listen to what they say without interrupting or making assumptions. Offer alternative methods of communication if needed and always be sensitive to their feelings. Educating ourselves about stuttering and maintaining a calm and positive attitude can create an inclusive and comfortable environment for effective communication.

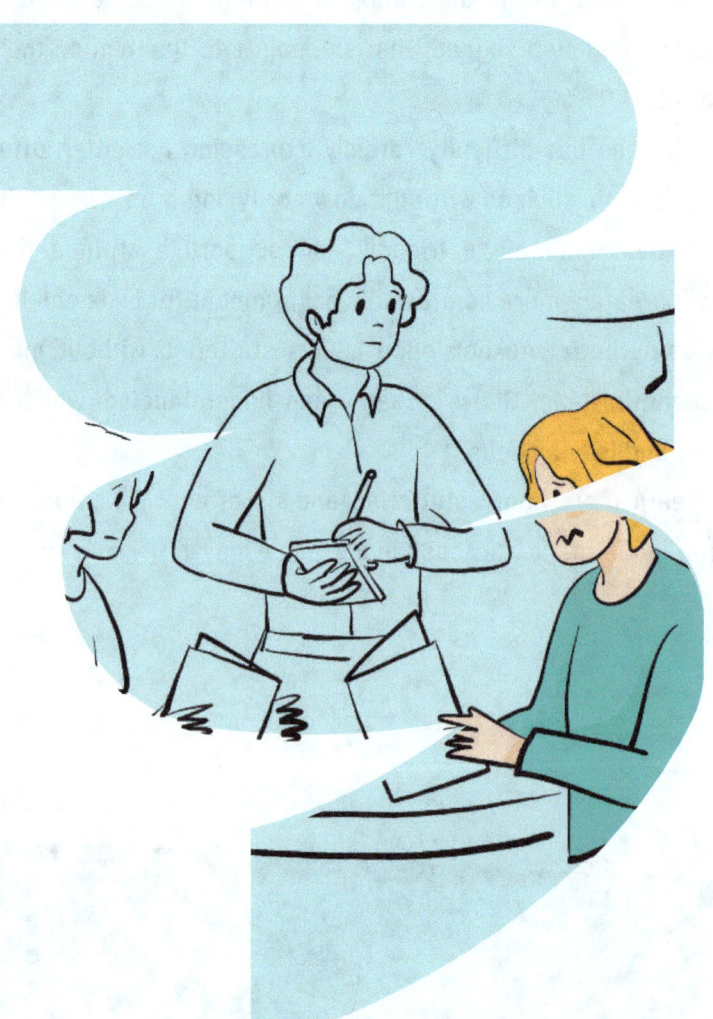

2

Story analysis

Questions...

1. On a scale of 1 to 10 (1 = very little, 10 = very much), how much do you think Lena stutters?

2. How did Lena feel when she had difficulty ordering food at the restaurant?

3. What thoughts passed Lena's mind when the waiter didn't understand her order?

4. Did Lena's friend offer Lena any support or help during the situation?

5. How might Lena's experience of stuttering affect her confidence in social situations?

6. Had Lena ever experienced a similar situation before? If so, how did she deal with it?

7. What strategies can Lena use to manage her stuttering in social situations, such as ordering food at a restaurant?

8. How might Lena's self-talk or internal dialogue affect her experience of stuttering in public?

9. How can Lena's friend be a supportive ally in situations where she may be struggling with her stuttering?

10. Are there activities or hobbies that Lena enjoys that make her feel less embarrassed about her stuttering?

3 A relaxed conversation

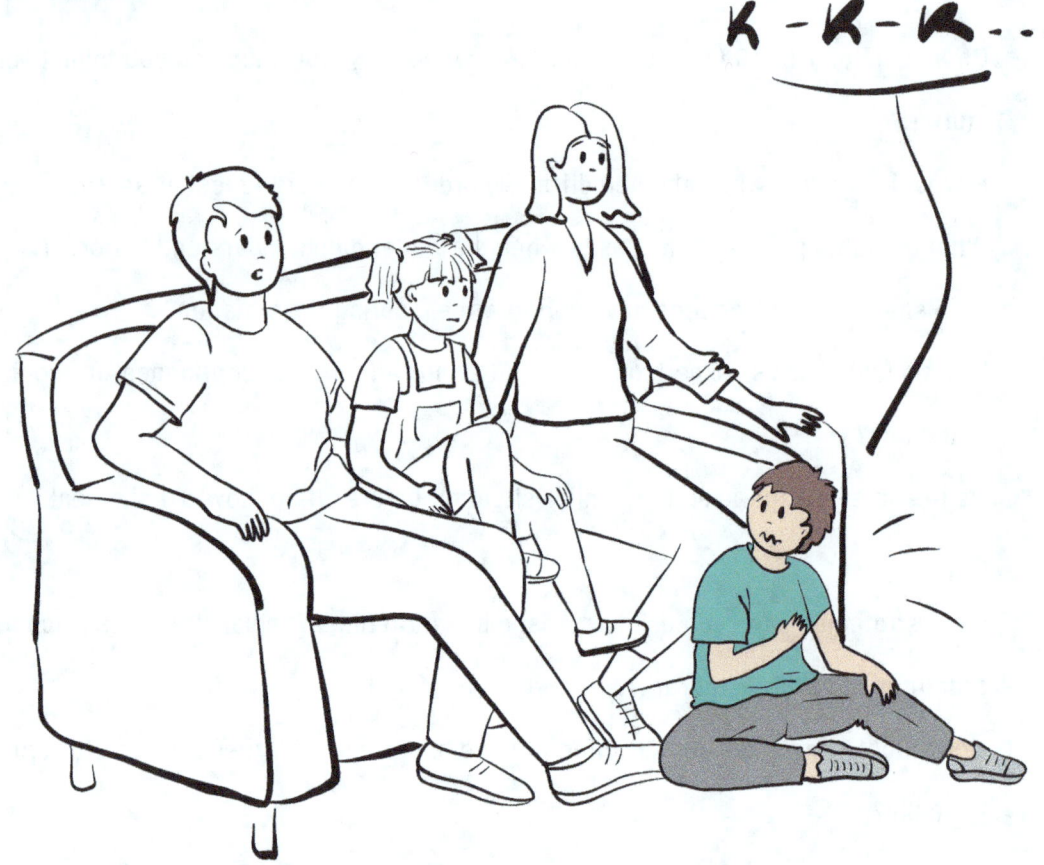

Sam, an eight-year-old stuttering child, hangs in the living room with his family. When his dad asks about his day at school, Sam feels a lump in his throat as he tries to form his answer. He can hear his heart pounding and feels awkward and uncomfortable.

Story analysis

From Sam's perspective

A. Thoughts and feelings:

Sam may feel...

- Anxiety and discomfort as he struggles to form words and speak fluently.
- Embarrassment or frustration about not being able to communicate effectively.

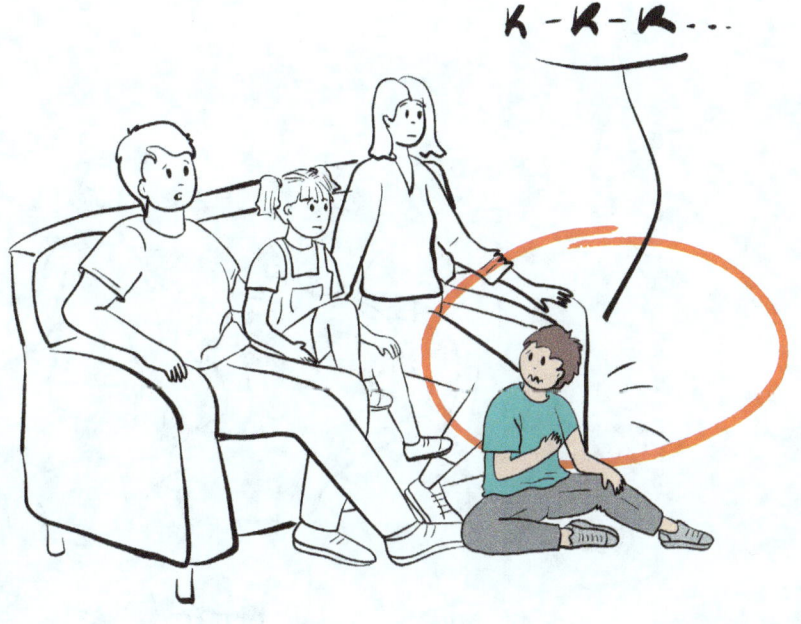

K-K-K-...

B. Possible actions:

- Sam may avoid eye contact, look down or get nervous.
- He may try to speak slowly and carefully or refrain from speaking completely.
- He may continue talking as if nothing is happening.

Story analysis

From the father's perspective

A. Thoughts and feelings:

The father may...

- Ignore Sam's stuttering and expect a typical reaction from his child.
- Feel surprised, confused, or worried when Sam has difficulty responding.

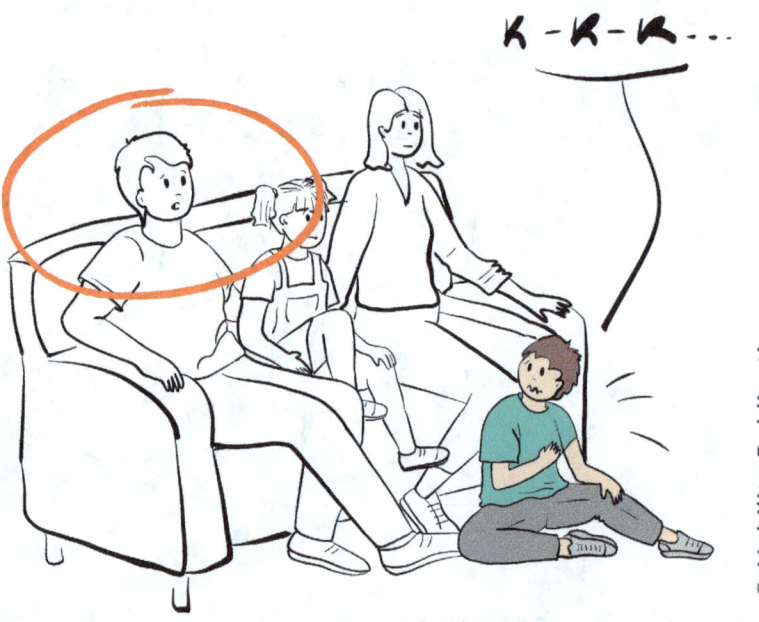

B. Possible actions:

- The father may try to help Sam by completing his sentences or speaking for him.
- He may offer encouragement or reassurance to help Sam feel more comfortable talking.
- He may stay calm and wait.

Story analysis

From the perspective of bystanders

A. Thoughts and feelings:

- Bystanders, who may be other family members or friends, may sympathize with Sam for his struggle with stuttering.
- They may also feel uncertain about how to react to the situation and become concerned about Sam's well-being.

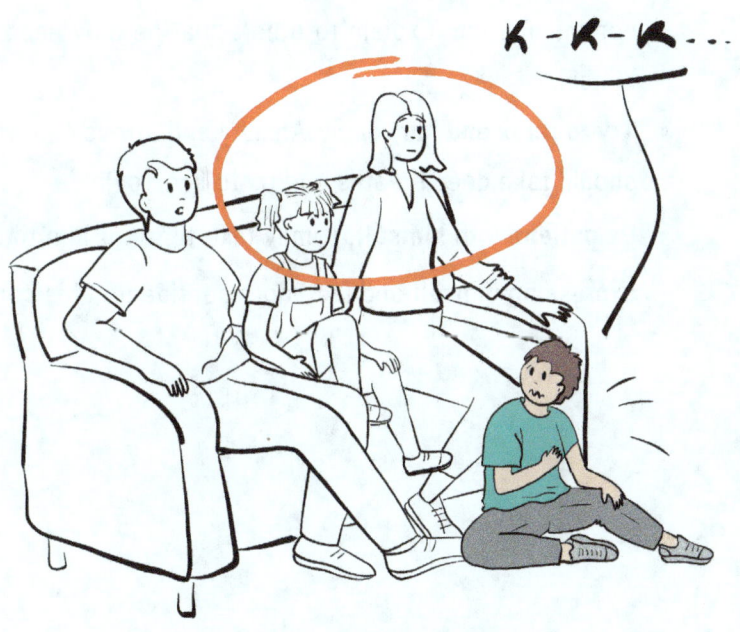

© Upbility Publications

B. Possible actions:

- Bystanders may offer emotional support to Sam or help facilitate the discussion by asking questions or providing additional context.
- They may try to create a comfortable and supportive environment that allows Sam to express himself freely.

Story analysis

Tips for effective communication:

Sam should:

- **Take his time and speak slowly:** Remember to take deep breaths, speak slowly, and not rush.
- **Use pauses:** Use short pauses to manage his speech better.
- **Be honest:** Be honest about his stuttering and how it affects his communication. Explain to others that he may need more time to express himself.
- **Try to relax and stay calm:** Anxiety and stress can worsen stuttering, so he should take deep breaths and try to keep calm.
- **Be patient with himself:** It may take time for him to get used to his way of expressing himself and feel more confident in his communication.

Story analysis

Tips for effective communication:

Sam's dad and other family members should:

- **Be patient and give Sam the time he needs to communicate:** Avoid interrupting him or completing his sentences.

- **Show interest in what he has to say:** Actively listen to him and encourage him to share his thoughts and feelings.

- **Not focus their attention on his stuttering:** Not focus on his disrupted speech, or ask too many questions about it unless he mentions it himself.

- **Be supportive and understanding:** Tell Sam they appreciate his efforts to communicate and are there for him.

- **Not make assumptions or criticisms based on his stuttering:** Remember that Sam struggles hard.

- **Create a comfortable and supportive environment:** Try to avoid a stressful or uncomfortable environment that may make Sam anxious.

- **Ask how they can help:** Ask Sam how they can help him communicate more effectively and try to accommodate his needs as best as possible.

Story analysis

Summary

Effective communication is a fundamental skill vital for building positive relationships, regardless of any speech problems or other obstacles. It's important to be patient, supportive, and understanding when communicating with someone with a speech disorder, such as stuttering, and to actively listen to what they say. By showing empathy, patience, and understanding, we can connect with others and create a more inclusive and supportive community.

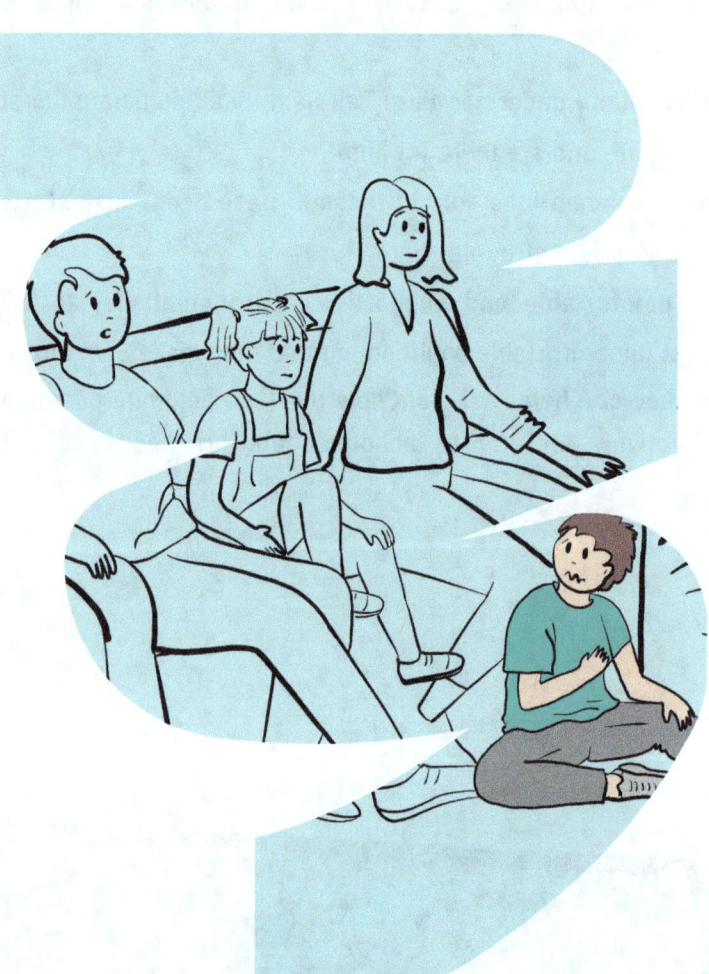

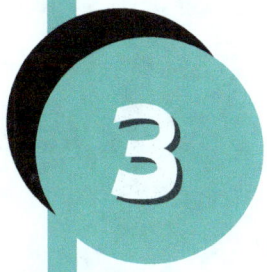

3

Story analysis

Questions...

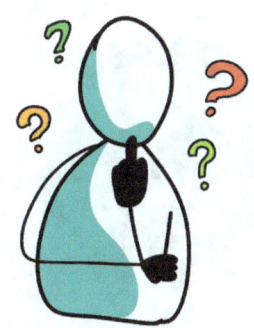

1. On a scale of 1 to 10 (1 = very little, 10 = very much), how much do you think Sam stutters?

2. What thoughts were going through Sam's mind when his dad asked him a question?

3. How did his body react when he tried to answer his dad's question?

4. What emotions did he experience at that moment?

5. Can you identify any negative thoughts or beliefs affecting you when you speak?

6. How could you change those negative thoughts or beliefs with more positive and realistic ones?

7. What coping techniques have you learned or practiced to manage your stuttering when you feel uncomfortable or nervous?

8. Can you think of any past experiences where you could speak without stuttering or with less stuttering that you could use to gain confidence?

9. What support is available to you at home, school, or elsewhere to help you manage your stuttering?

10. How could Sam communicate with his father and other family members about his stuttering so that they can understand and support him better?

4 An important conversation

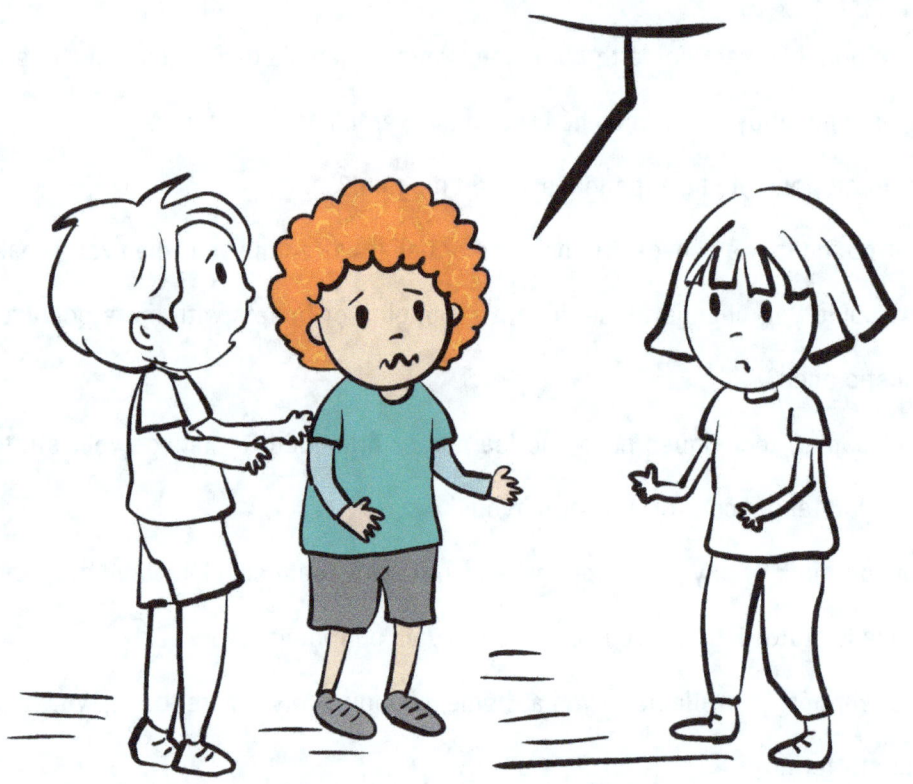

mo - mo - mo ...

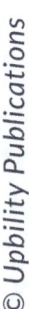
One day in the schoolyard, Penny discusses something important with her friends. Penny tries to explain something, but her stuttering makes her friends impatient. As she struggles with speaking, she realizes that stress and frustration are making it even worse.

Story analysis

From Penny's perspective

A. Thoughts and feelings:

Penny feels extremely anxious and embarrassed about her stuttering. She becomes increasingly frustrated with herself as she tries to explain something important to her friends. She senses their impatience and feels even more pressure to communicate her thoughts clearly. This intensifies her anxiety, making her stuttering even worse. Penny feels embarrassed, hurt, and isolated.

mo - mo - mo ...

B. Possible actions:

- Penny could take a deep breath, pause for a moment and try to calm down before attempting to speak again.
- She could use alternative communication methods, such as writing down her thoughts or using gestures.
- She could also talk to a close friend about her feelings and ask for their understanding and patience.
- Alternatively, she could seek professional help, such as speech therapy, to improve her stuttering and boost her confidence.

Story analysis

From the friend's perspective

A. Thoughts and feelings:

Penny's friend may feel...

- Sympathy for her and worry about her struggle to communicate.
- Anger or frustration towards their other friends for not being more understanding and patient. He wants to support Penny and make her feel better.

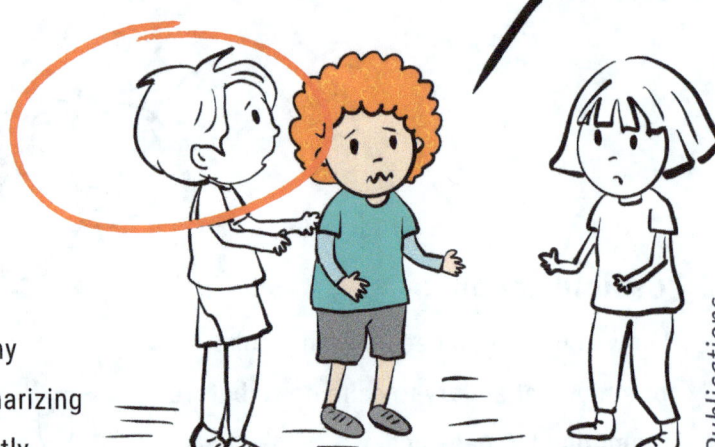

mo - mo - mo ...

B. Possible actions:

- He could step in and help Penny express her thoughts by summarizing what she's trying to say or gently prompting her when she gets stuck.
- He could pull Penny aside, console her and offer words of encouragement.
- He could also reach out to their friends, reminding them to be patient and understanding while Penny talks.
- Later, he could discuss with Penny the possibility of seeking professional help or joining a support group for people who stutter.

Story analysis

From the perspective of bystanders

A. Thoughts and feelings:

- Bystanders may feel various emotions, from sympathy and concern for Penny to anticipation of hearing her thoughts or even the impulse to be amused by her struggle.

- Some may feel uncomfortable by the situation, while others may want to help but be unsure about what to do.

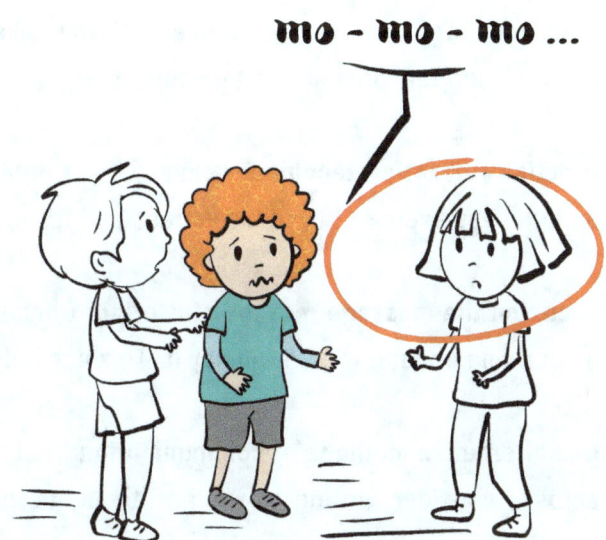

B. Possible actions:

- Bystanders could choose to intervene, offering Penny their support and encouraging her friends to be more patient.

- They could also simply offer her a friendly smile or a reassuring look to let her know they understand and sympathize with her situation.

- On the other hand, some bystanders may choose to ignore the situation or even laugh at Penny's expense.

- Others may decide to talk about the incident with their friends or family later, spreading awareness about stuttering and the need for patience and understanding.

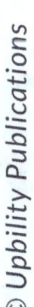

Story analysis

Tips for effective communication:

Penny should:

Take her time: Allow herself to speak slowly, take deep breaths, and pause when needed. Not rush and feel pressure to talk quickly.

Practice relaxation techniques: Learn deep breathing, progressive muscle relaxation, or mindfulness exercises to reduce stress and tension when speaking.

Focus on the message, not the stuttering: Concentrate on what she wants to say instead of worrying about how she will say it. This can help reduce anxiety and stress.

Use alternative methods of communication: If she is having difficulty getting her message across, consider writing down her thoughts or using gestures to communicate her message.

Seek professional help: Consider working with a speech and language therapist to develop strategies and techniques to deal with stuttering.

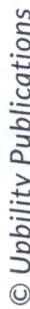

© Upbility Publications

Story analysis

Tips for effective communication:

Penny's friends should:

Be patient: Give Penny plenty of time to express herself and avoid finishing her sentences or interrupting her. This will help her feel more relaxed and supported.

Maintain eye contact: Make sure they maintain eye contact and show active listening, which can help Penny to feel more comfortable and confident while talking.

Avoid drawing attention to stuttering: Avoid pointing out the stuttering or making jokes about it. Instead, focus on the content of the conversation.

Offer encouragement: Offer reassurance and support, letting Penny know they understand her struggle and are there to help.

Educate themselves: Learn more about stuttering and the challenges faced by people who stutter. This will help them better understand and empathize with Penny's situation.

Become her allies: Encourage others to be patient and understanding when communicating with Penny and address any misunderstandings or nasty comments about stuttering.

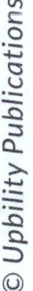

© Upbility Publications

Story analysis

Summary

Effective communication is vital for building strong relationships and promoting understanding between individuals. For both Penny and her friends, it's important to practice patience, empathy, and active listening. Penny can benefit from adopting relaxation techniques, focusing on her message, and considering alternative methods of communication. Meanwhile, her friends can support her by maintaining eye contact, offering encouragement, and learning about stuttering. By working together, Penny and her friends can foster an inclusive environment where everyone's voice is valued and heard. Let's not forget that communication is a two-way street, and it takes effort from both parties to ensure a successful and meaningful exchange of ideas.

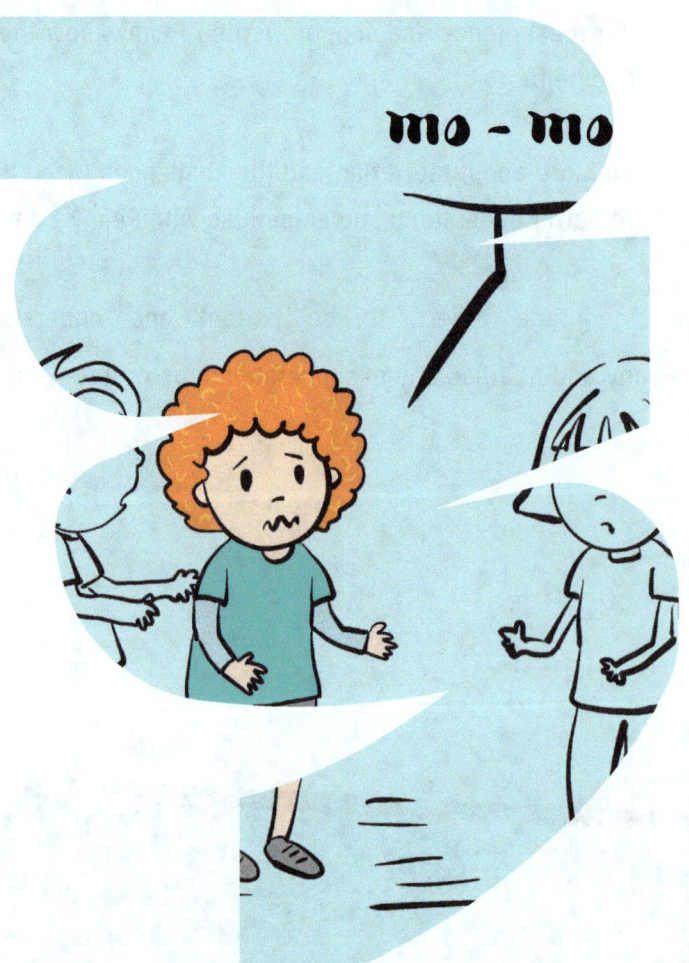

© Upbility Publications

Story analysis

Questions...

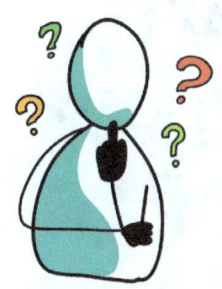

1. On a scale of 1 to 10 (1 = very little, 10 = very much), how much do you think Penny stutters?

2. How did Penny feel when her friends became impatient with her stuttering?

3. What thoughts do you think Penny might have had while struggling to communicate with her friends?

4. Have you ever experienced something similar where you felt judged or misunderstood because of your stuttering?

5. In this case, what might be some helpful coping strategies that Penny could use to manage her stuttering?

6. How might practicing relaxation techniques like deep breathing or slow speech help Penny manage her stuttering?

7. What are some positive things Penny's friends could do to support her when she stutters?

8. How can Penny communicate her needs to her friends when she has difficulty speaking?

9. Have you ever talked with someone about how they can support you when you stutter?

10. How can positive self-talk help Penny manage her frustration and anxiety when she stutters?

11. Have you ever tried a speech therapy technique, such as controlled pauses, to manage your stuttering in social situations?

5 A new friend

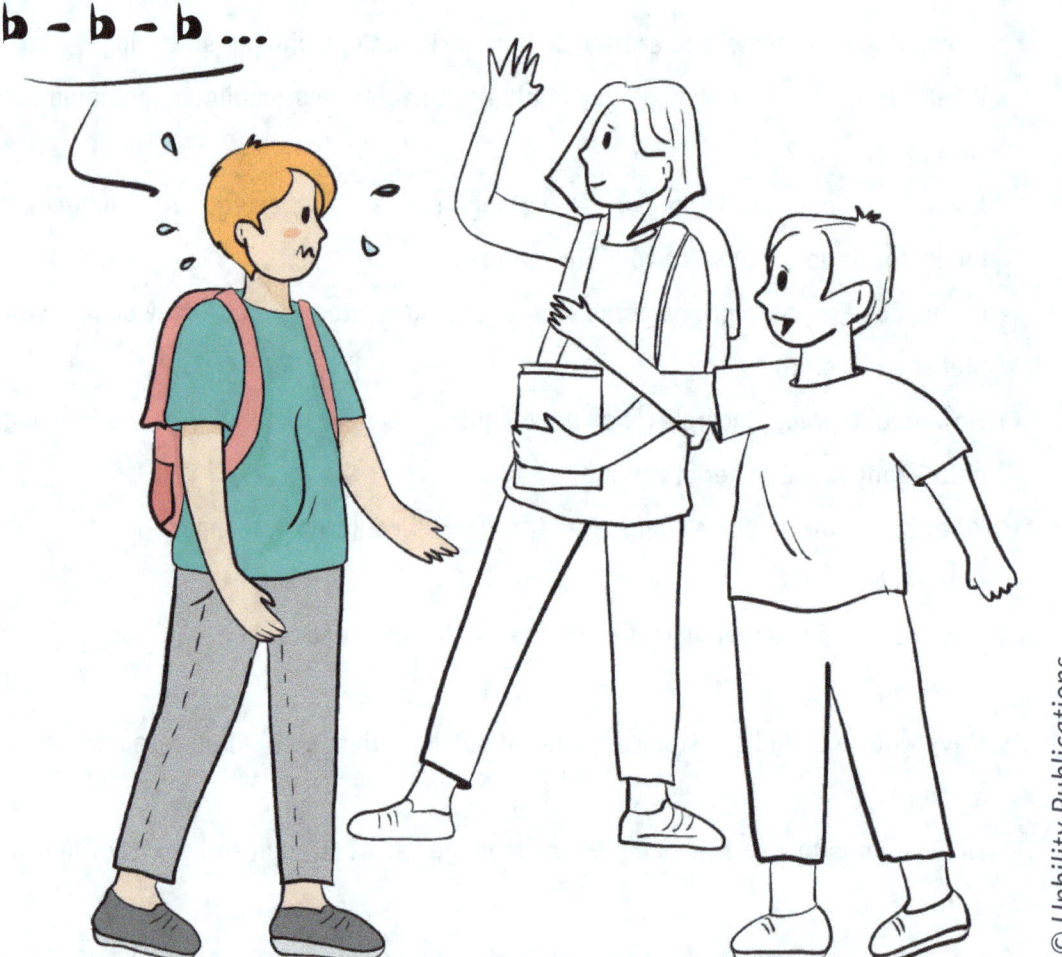

Jim tries to introduce himself to a new friend, but his stuttering makes it difficult, resulting in embarrassment and confusion.

5 Story analysis

From Jim's perspective

A. Thoughts and feelings:

Jim may feel...

- Anxious about what his new friend will think.
- Sad or frustrated that his speech disorder will keep him from making a good first impression.

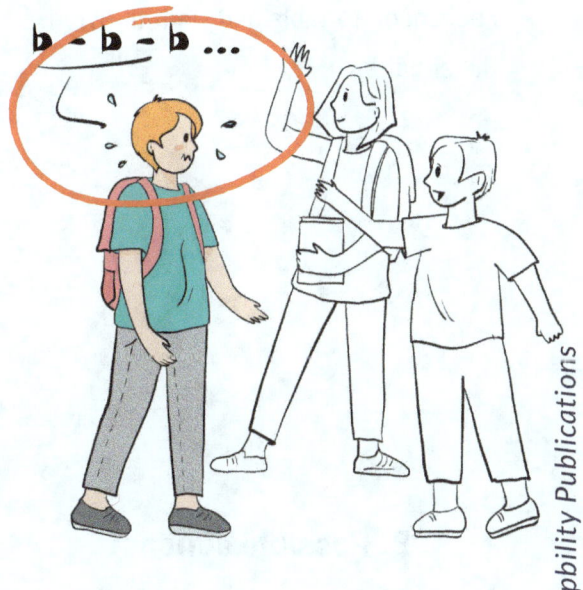

B. Possible actions:

- Jim may avoid speaking completely or keep his interactions with the new friend to a minimum to avoid further embarrassment.
- Alternatively, he may try to overcome his stuttering and continue to introduce himself despite the difficulties he is experiencing.

Story analysis

From the new friend's perspective

A. Thoughts and feelings:

The new friend may...

- Feel confused or uncertain about how to react to Jim's stuttering and sympathize with his struggles.
- Be curious to learn more about his stuttering.
- Feel uncomfortable and want to avoid the situation.

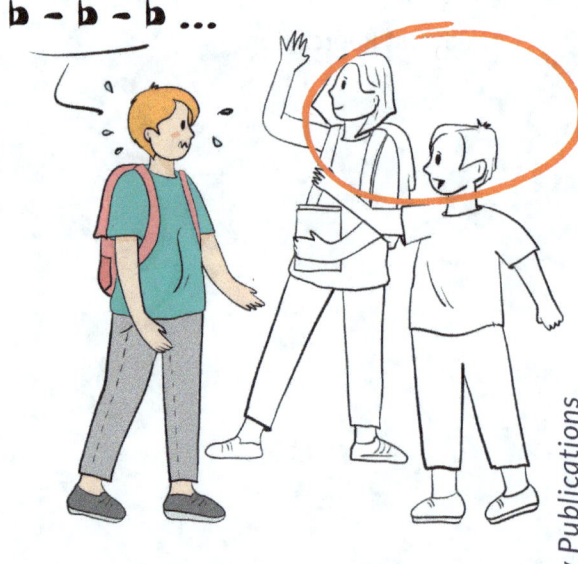

B. Possible actions:

- The new friend may try to actively listen and have a conversation with Jim or not know how to respond and try to conclude their conversation quickly.
- He may also ask questions about Jim's stuttering to understand the situation better.

Story analysis

From the perspective of bystanders

A. Thoughts and feelings:

- Bystanders may feel sympathy for Jim and his struggle with stuttering.
- They may be uncomfortable and unsure how to react to the situation.
- They may also feel frustrated or annoyed if the conversation becomes awkward or tense.

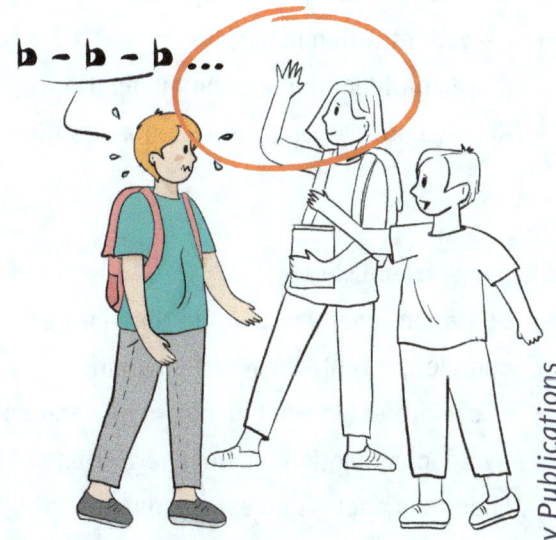

B. Possible actions:

- Bystanders may try to intervene and help facilitate the discussion.
- They may try to ignore the situation entirely.
- They may try to provide emotional support to Jim or the new friend, depending on their personal feelings about the situation.

Story analysis

Tips for effective communication:

Jim should:

- Be honest about his stuttering and how it affects his communication. Explain that he may need more time to express himself.
- Use strategies such as slow and soft speech, breath control, and pauses to manage his stuttering.
- Try to relax and remain calm. Anxiety and stress can worsen stuttering, so he should take deep breaths and stay calm.
- Be patient with himself. It may take time to become familiar with a new friend and feel more confident in their communication.
- Receive professional help from a qualified speech and language therapist.

Jim's new friend should:

- Be patient and give Jim the time he needs to communicate. Avoid interrupting him or completing sentences on his behalf.
- Show interest in what he has to say and actively listen to him.
- Avoid commenting on his new friend's speech difficulty or asking him too many questions about it unless he mentions it himself.
- Be supportive and show understanding. Show Jim that he appreciates his efforts to communicate and that he is there for him.
- Not make assumptions or criticisms based on his stuttering. Remember that his new friend is struggling.

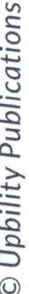

Story analysis

Summary

For Jim, it can be difficult to introduce himself to a new friend because of his stuttering. Still, he can overcome his anxiety by believing in himself and being patient. On the other hand, Jim's new friend must be patient, supportive, and understanding. Also, avoid unnecessary attention to Jim's stuttering and actively listen to what he says.

In conclusion, effective communication is critical to building positive relationships, regardless of any speech problems or other obstacles. By showing empathy, patience, and understanding, we can connect with others and create a more inclusive and supportive community.

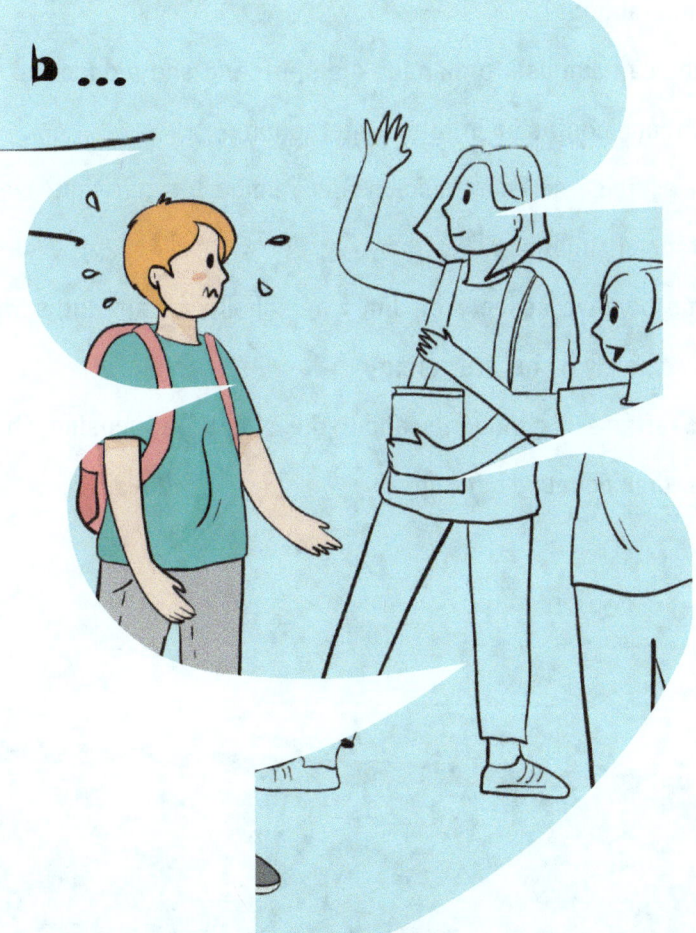

5

Story analysis

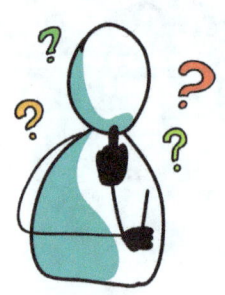

Questions...

1. On a scale of 1 to 10 (1 = very little, 10 = very much), how much do you think Jim stutters?

2. What thoughts were going through Jim's mind as he introduced himself to the new friend?

3. How did Jim feel when he began to stutter during his speech?

4. What emotions did Jim experience as a result of the embarrassment and confusion?

5. What were some things the new friend might have thought or felt during their conversation?

6. How did the situation affect Jim's confidence and willingness to participate in future social interactions?

7. What strategies can Jim use to manage his stuttering and reduce the likelihood of embarrassment and confusion in future interactions?

8. How can Jim exercise self-compassion and remind himself that everyone faces challenges in social situations?

9. What are some positive aspects of Jim's personality or strengths where he can focus instead of solely on his stuttering?

10. How can Jim reframe his thoughts about the situation, focusing on growth and learning rather than negative outcomes?

Visiting a friend

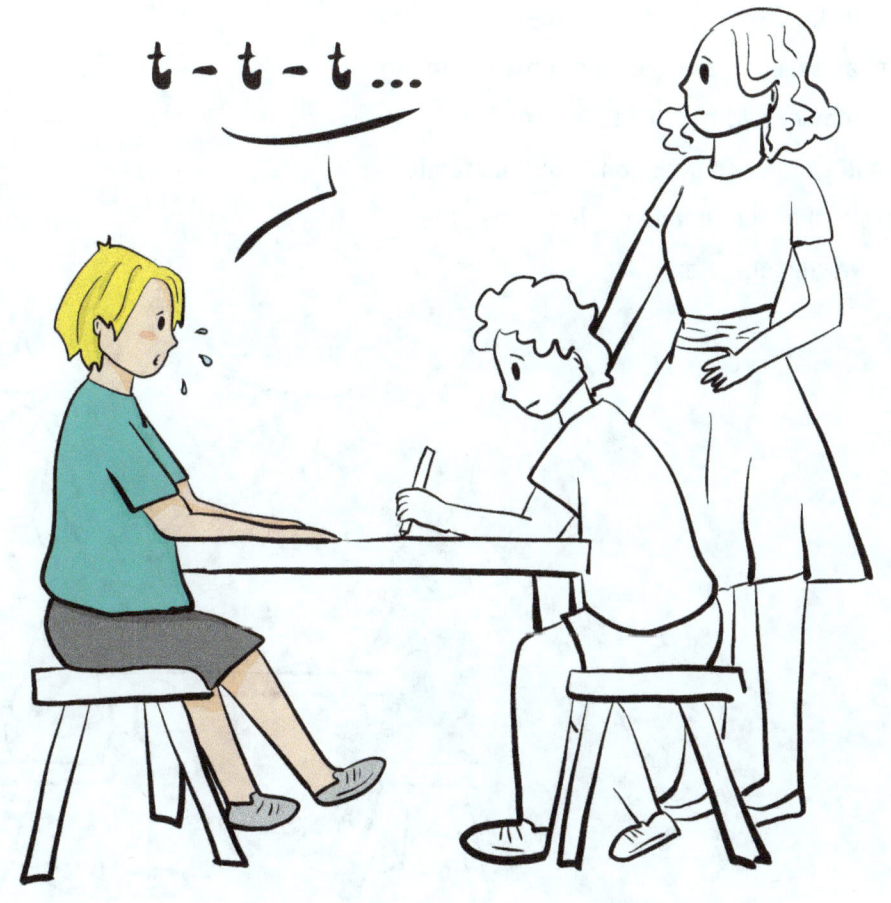

Bo visits his friend's house to work on a school project together. When his friend's mother asks how his family is doing, Bo has a hard time answering because of his stuttering.

Story analysis

From Bo's perspective

A. Thoughts and feelings:

Bo may feel...

- Embarrassed or anxious about his stuttering and may have difficulty answering his friend's mother's question about his family.
- Afraid, thinking that he might not be able to answer the question.

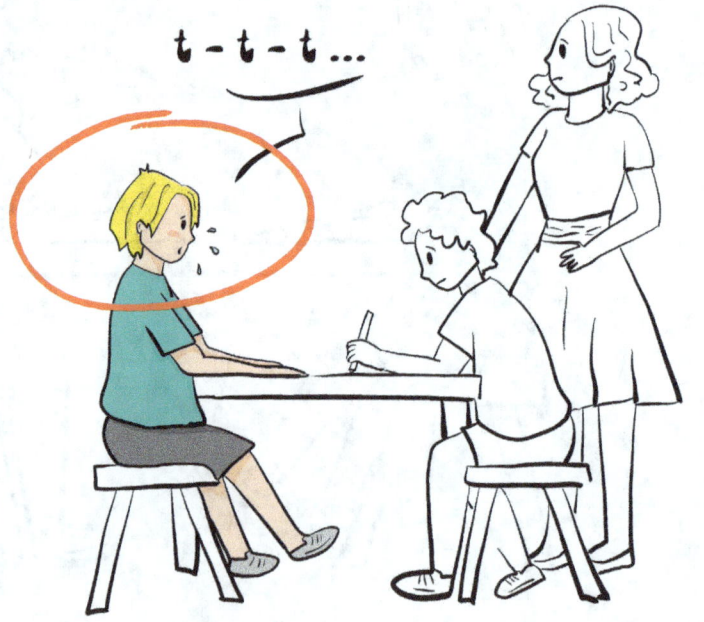

B. Possible actions:

- He may try to avoid the issue or get frustrated if he cannot communicate effectively.
- He may be brief in his response.
- He may respond properly, trying not to think about his stuttering.

Story analysis

From his friend's mother's perspective

A. Thoughts and feelings:

His friend's mother may...

- Be concerned about Bo's family and want to open up a conversation.
- Feel unsure or uncomfortable with Bo's stuttering and may not know how to react.

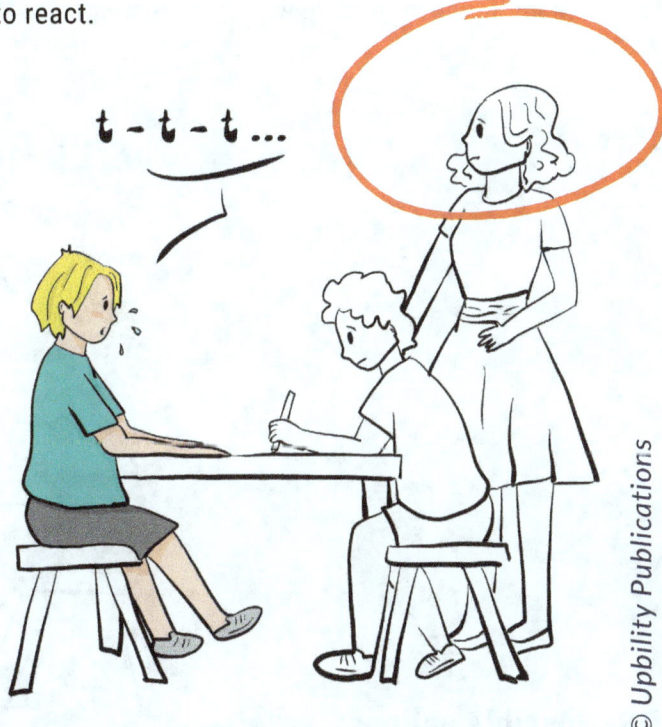

t - t - t...

© Upbility Publications

B. Possible actions:

- His friend's mother may try to offer reassurance and support to Bo. For example, by saying something like "It's okay, take your time," or changing the conversation.
- Alternatively, she may unintentionally make Bo more uncomfortable by trying to complete his sentences or interrupting him.
- She may remain calm and wait patiently for Bo to complete his sentence.

Story analysis

From the perspective of bystanders

A. Thoughts and feelings:

- Bystanders may feel sympathy for Bo and empathize with his difficulty in communicating.
- They may also feel uncertain about how to react or uncomfortable with the situation.

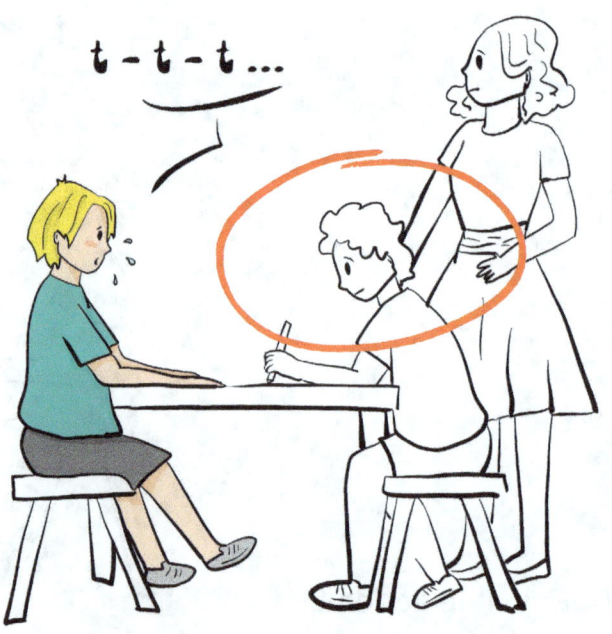

t - t - t...

© Upbility Publications

B. Possible actions:

- Bystanders can offer support to Bo by letting him take his time or changing the subject. They can also provide encouragement or positive feedback to boost Bo's confidence.
- Alternatively, they may avoid the situation or try to ignore the problem.

Story analysis

Tips for effective communication:

Be patient: It's important to be patient and give Bo the time he needs to talk. Pressuring him or completing his sentences can make him feel more anxious and embarrassed.

Avoid interrupting him: If you interrupt Bo as he struggles to speak, he may become frustrated and discouraged. Wait for him to finish before you respond.

Show interest: Show interest in what Bo says and let him know that you are listening. This can help him feel more comfortable and gain more confidence.

Don't focus on stuttering: Try not to focus on Bo's stuttering or make it the main topic of conversation. Instead, focus on what he says.

Use non-verbal cues: Use non-verbal cues such as nodding, maintaining eye contact, and smiling to show you are engaged and supportive.

Do not give unsolicited advice: Unless Bo asks for advice on improving his speech, avoid giving it, as this can be counterproductive and make him feel more embarrassed.

Be supportive: Encourage and support Bo in his efforts to communicate. Recognize his strengths and help him feel respected and valued.

Remember, effective communication is a two-way street; both parties must work together to succeed. You can help Bo feel more confident and comfortable communicating with you with patience, support, and understanding.

Story analysis

Summary

Effective communication is essential for building relationships, achieving goals, and promoting understanding. When communicating with someone who stutters, it's important to be patient, supportive, and compassionate. Stuttering can be a frustrating and upsetting experience, and it is crucial to create a safe and welcoming environment that encourages open and honest communication. Using these tips, we can help people who stutter feel more confident and comfortable communicating and create meaningful connections that foster understanding and appreciation for each other.

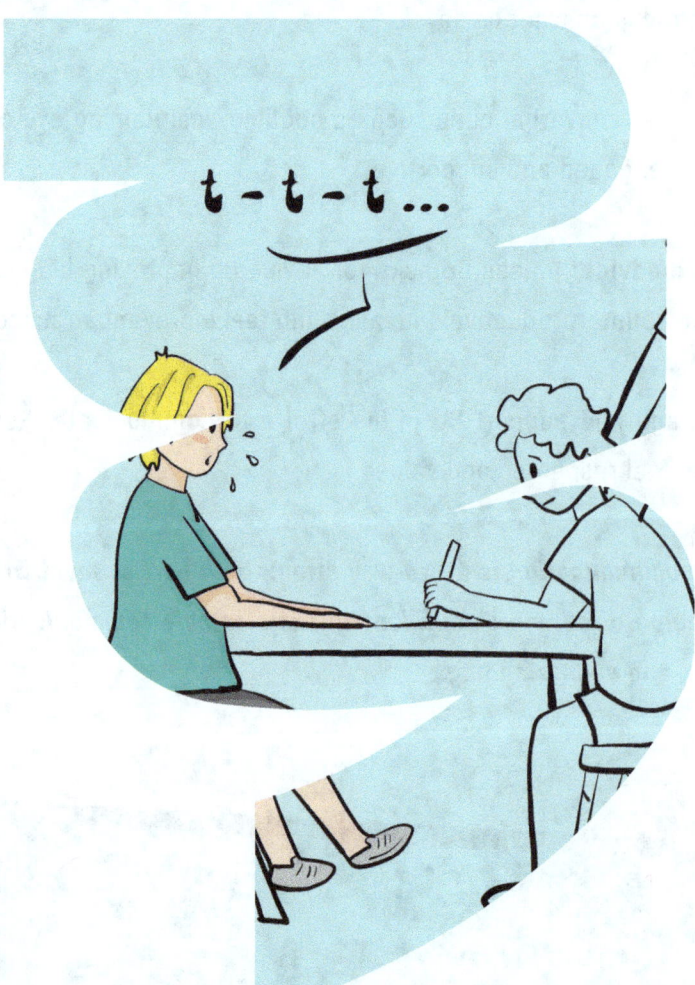

6

Story analysis

Questions...

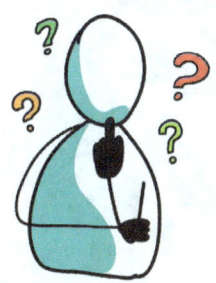

1. On a scale of 1 to 10 (1 = very little, 10 = very much), how much do you think Bo stutters?

2. How does Bo feel about his stuttering when he talks to his friend's mother?

3. What thoughts go through Bo's mind when asked about his family?

4. Can Bo identify specific triggers or situations that worsen his stuttering?

5. How does Bo's stuttering affect his ability to complete the school project with his friend?

6. What coping strategies has Bo used in the past to deal with his stuttering?

7. How would Bo feel if he could respond to his friend's mother without stuttering?

8. Can Bo think of any positive aspects of his stuttering or how it has helped him develop resilience or other skills?

9. How would Bo describe his support system, and who can he turn to when he feels anxious or upset about his stuttering?

10. What small steps can Bo take to improve his communication and gain confidence despite his stuttering?

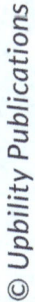

7 The disagreement

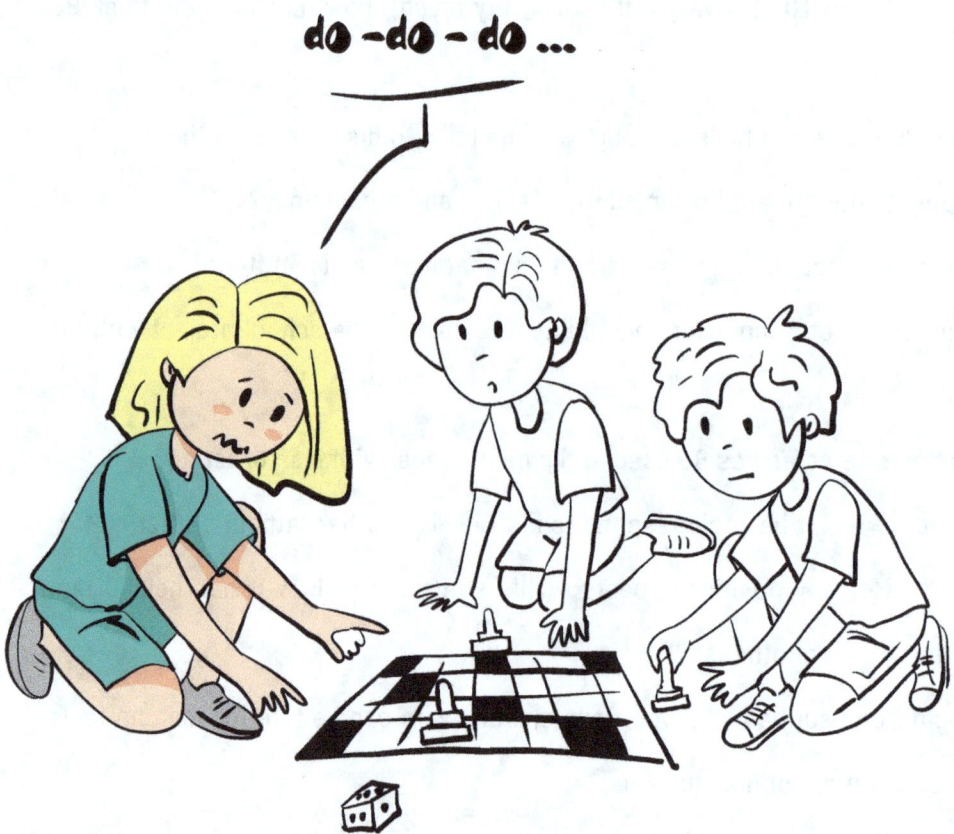

do -do - do ...

© Upbility Publications

Stella and her friends are playing a game in the schoolyard. As they discuss the rules, they argue with each other. Stella wants to speak her mind, but her words get stuck. She struggles to speak, and her friends become impatient, thinking she is nervous. In the end, one of the children interrupts her and rejects her idea. Stella feels embarrassed and upset. She wonders if she will ever be able to speak her mind without stuttering.

Story analysis

From Stella's perspective

A. Thoughts and feelings:

Stella may...

- Feel frustrated and embarrassed because she found it difficult to speak, and her friends became impatient with her.
- Wonder if she'll ever be able to speak her mind without stuttering.

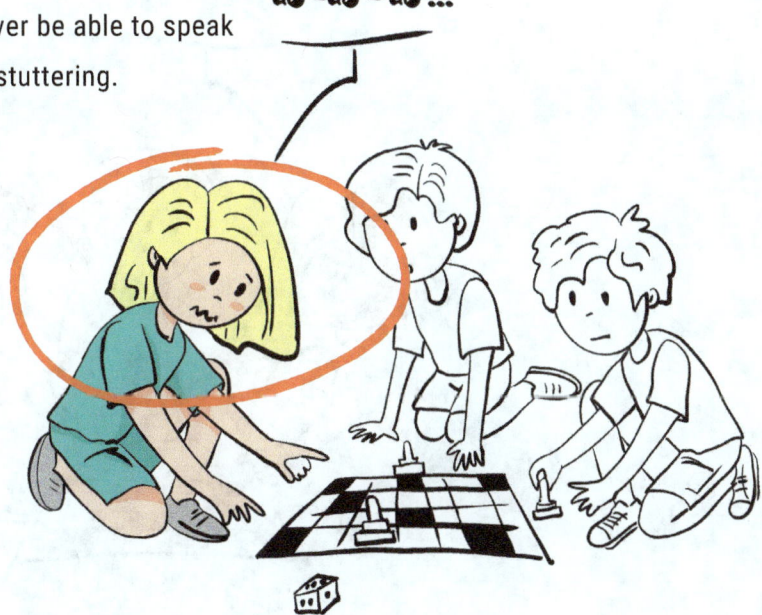

B. Possible actions:

- Stella may feel discouraged and hesitate to speak in the future.
- She may try to work on her speech disorder and find ways to overcome it.

Story analysis

From the perspective of the child who interrupted Stella

A. Thoughts and feelings:

The child who interrupted Stella may:

- Feel that she was too slow to express herself and that her idea could wait.
- Think that Stella was just nervous and not confident enough to speak.

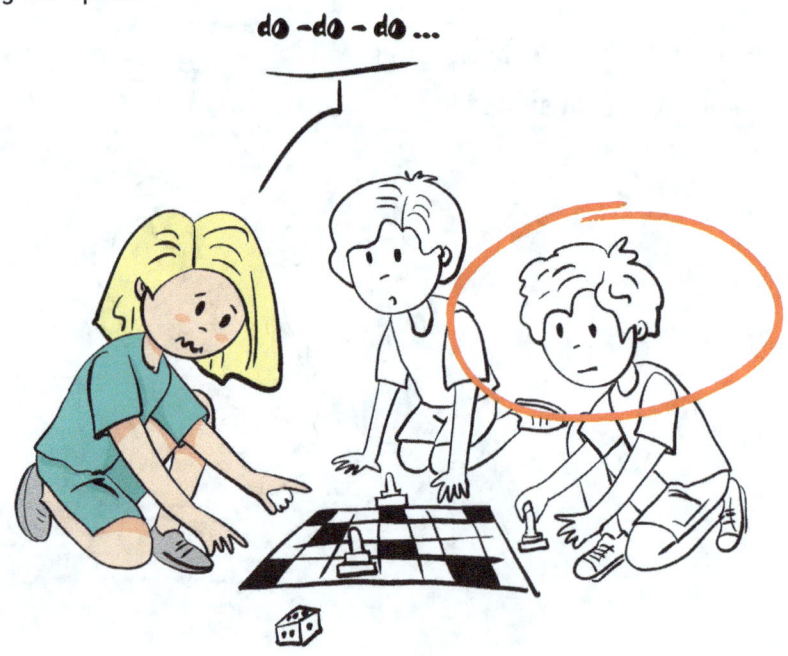

B. Possible actions:

- The child may keep rejecting Stella's ideas in the future, remaining unaware of her condition.
- The child may become more patient and understanding of her speech difficulty.

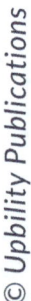

Story analysis

From the perspective of bystanders

A. Thoughts and feelings:

- Bystanders may feel uncomfortable with Stella's disagreement and subsequent struggle to speak.
- They may also feel impatient and frustrated about the situation.

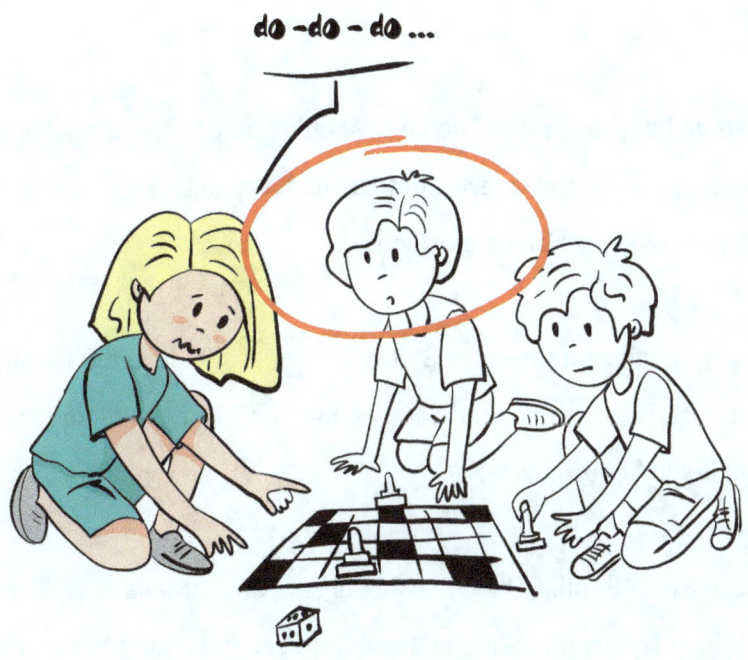

do -do - do ...

B. Possible actions:

- Bystanders can try to intervene and encourage everyone to listen to each other's ideas.
- They can also support Stella and help her feel more comfortable speaking up in the future.
- They may even stand by and not take sides in the children's argument.

Story analysis

Tips for effective communication:

Be patient: The child should try to be patient with Stella's speech difficulty and give her enough time to express her thoughts.

Listen actively: The child should listen to what Stella is saying and try to understand her point of view. Interrupting her will increase her anxiety and prevent effective communication.

Use positive body language: The child should use positive body language to show interest and attention. Maintaining eye contact, nodding, and smiling can help Stella relax and encourage her to communicate effectively.

Avoid completing sentences for Stella: The child should avoid finishing Stella's sentences as this can be frustrating and undermine her confidence. Instead, they should let her finish her thoughts at her own pace.

Encourage Stella to talk: The child should encourage Stella to talk and share her ideas and offer positive feedback when she does. This can help build her confidence and encourage effective communication.

Show respect: The child should show respect and consideration for Stella and avoid making negative comments about her disfluency. This can help create a supportive and understanding environment for effective communication.

Story analysis

Summary

Stella's stuttering can be challenging, but she can overcome it with patience, understanding, and support. Those communicating with Stella should be patient, actively listen, use positive body language, avoid interrupting her or finishing her sentences, encourage her to speak, and respect her. It's also vital to create a supportive environment where Stella feels comfortable expressing herself without fear of criticism. By using these strategies, Stella can gain confidence and develop effective communication skills that will benefit her in all aspects of her life. Finally, it is important to remember that stuttering does not determine a person's intelligence or abilities and that everyone deserves to be heard and understood.

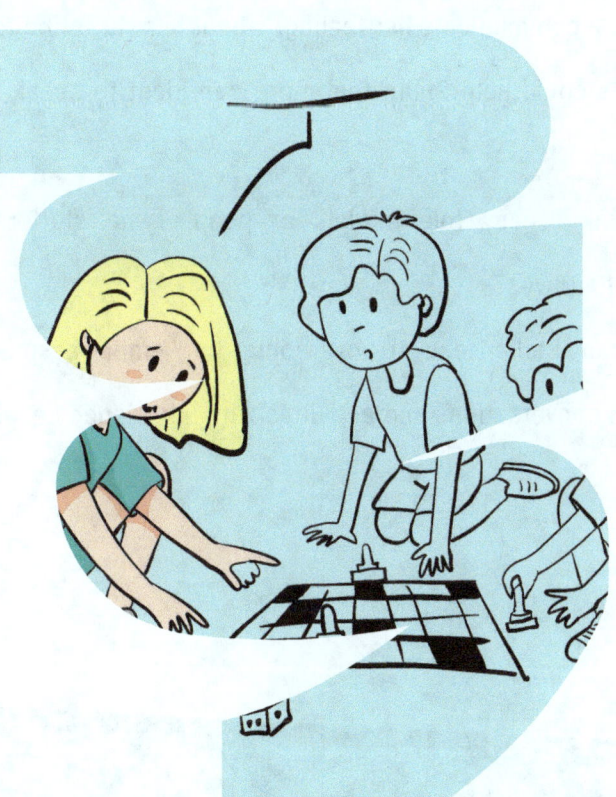

© Upbility Publications

7 Story analysis

Questions...

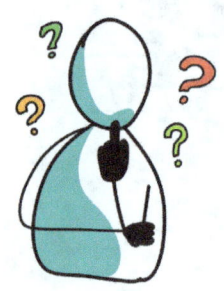

1. On a scale of 1 to 10 (1 = very little, 10 = very much), how much do you think Stella stutters?

2. How did Stella feel when her friends became impatient with her stuttering?

3. What thoughts went through Stella's mind when they interrupted and rejected her idea?

4. Can Stella think of any positive aspects or advantages she has, even though she stutters?

5. How might Stella's friends have reacted differently if they understood more about stuttering?

6. How can Stella practice speaking her mind, even though she stutters?

7. How could Stella communicate her feelings about her stuttering to her friends?

8. What strategies could help Stella feel more confident to speak up, even with her stuttering?

9. Can Stella think of any role models or people who stuttered and yet were successful in their lives?

10. What steps can Stella take to overcome her embarrassment and continue participating in conversations and activities with her friends despite her stuttering?

Family shopping

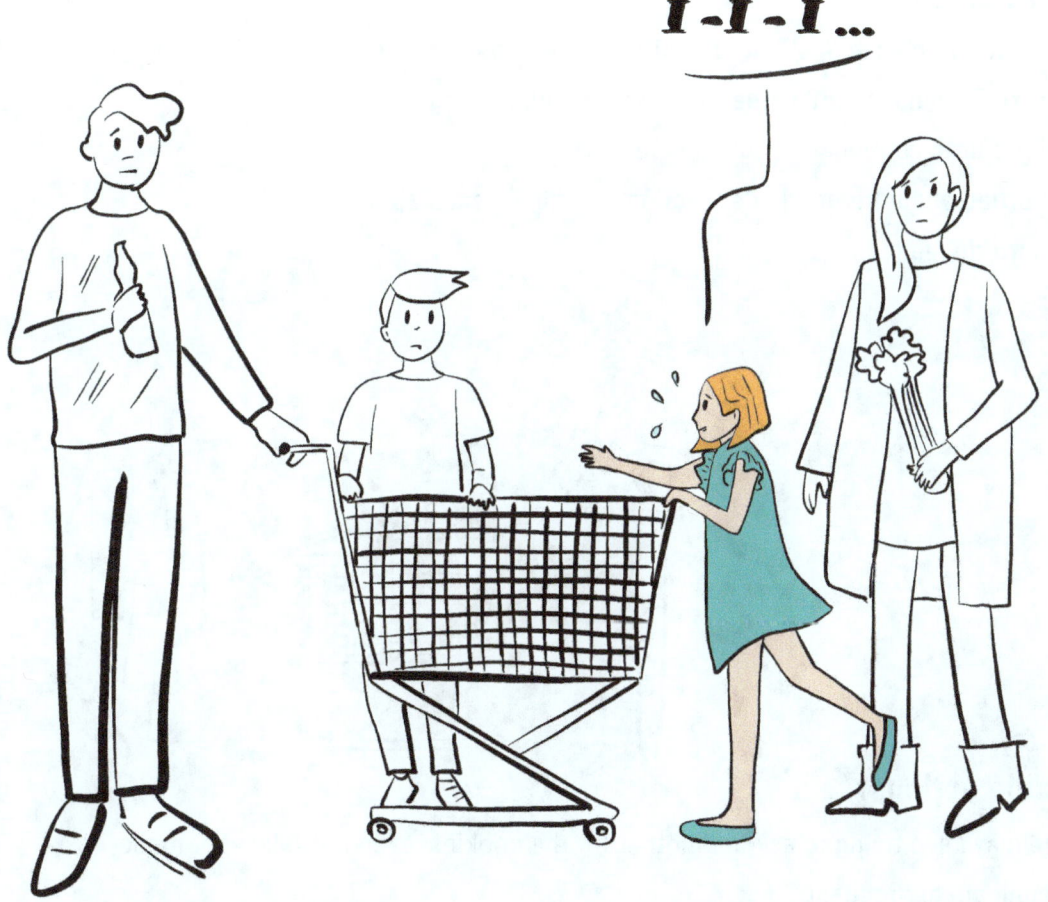

Sophie, a seven-year-old girl, visits the nearby supermarket with her family. On a high shelf, she spots her favorite cookies. She tries to ask her mother for help but finds it very hard because she stutters.

Story analysis

From Sophie's perspective

A. Thoughts and feelings:

Sophie may feel...

- Excited when she spots her favorite cookies on the shelf.
- Anxious and frustrated due to her stuttering, making it difficult to communicate her desire.
- Worried about her mother's reaction or embarrassed about stuttering in public.

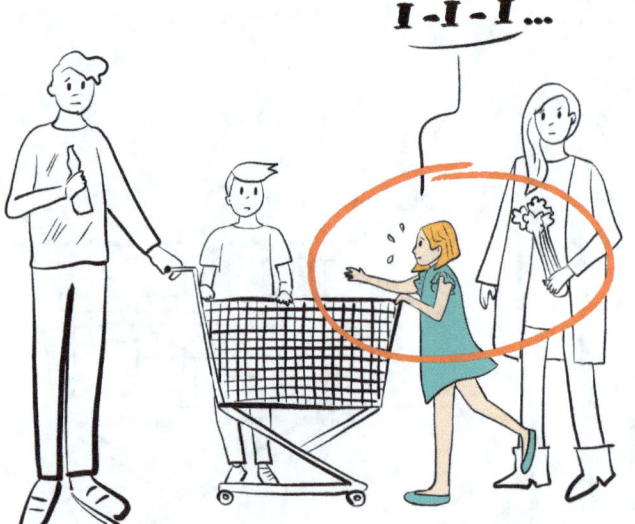

B. Possible actions:

- Sophie may keep trying to ask her mother for the cookies, even if it takes her longer to communicate her request.
- She may use alternative means of communication, such as pointing to the cookies or using gestures to express what she wants.
- Sophie may also try to suppress her desire and decide not to ask her mother for the cookies to avoid possible embarrassment or disappointment.

8 Story analysis

From the mother's perspective

A. Thoughts and feelings:

Sophie's mother may...

- Be concerned about Sophie's stuttering and difficulty communicating.
- Feel empathy for Sophie's struggle and worry about her daughter's possible embarrassment or discomfort in public.

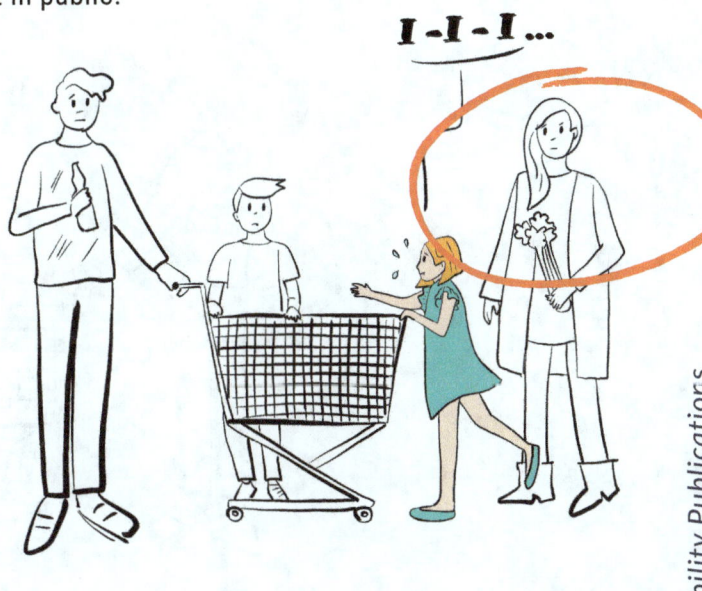

I-I-I...

B. Possible actions:

- Sophie's mother could acknowledge her daughter's struggle and ask if she wants the cookies.
- She could patiently listen to Sophie's request, offering encouragement and support as she tried to communicate.
- She could work with Sophie to develop her communication skills and seek professional help to cope with stuttering.

Story analysis

From the perspective of bystanders

A. Thoughts and feelings:

* Bystanders may feel curious or sympathetic, watching Sophie's struggle.
* Some may empathize with her and her mother, while others may not understand the situation or be uninterested.

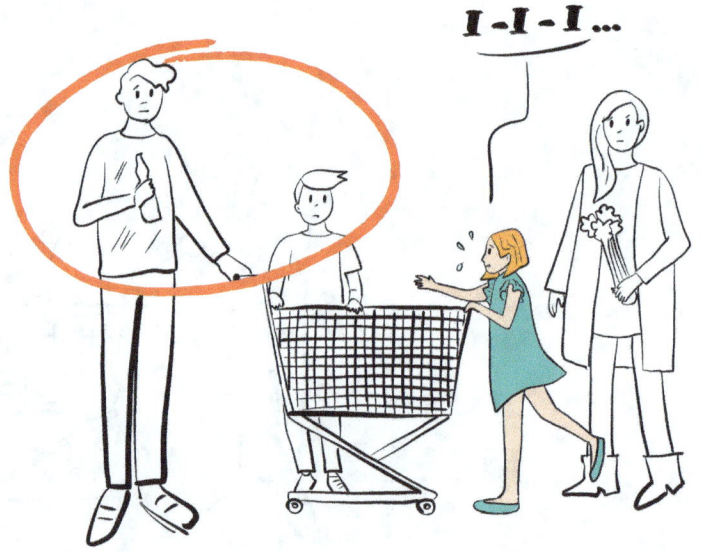

B. Possible actions:

* Bystanders may offer help, such as grabbing the cookies from the high shelf if they notice Sophie's desire.
* They could give Sophie and her mother space and privacy, allowing them to process the situation without additional pressure.
* Alternatively, some bystanders could offer uncalled advice or comments, which could be unhelpful or even harmful to Sophie's self-esteem and confidence.

Story analysis

Tips for effective communication:

Sophie should:

Use deep breathing and relaxation techniques: Calming the body and mind can help Sophie manage stress or anxiety associated with stuttering, facilitating communication.

Speak slowly and consciously: Taking time to pronounce each word carefully can help Sophie reduce the frequency of her stuttering.

Use alternative forms of communication: If speaking becomes too difficult, Sophie can use gestures, body language, or even texting to express herself.

Create conditions to increase confidence: It's good for Sophie to practice speaking in comforting and supportive environments to build her confidence and gradually become more comfortable in public situations.

Seek professional help: A speech and language therapist can work with Sophie to develop strategies and exercises to help her manage her stuttering.

Story analysis

Tips for effective communication:

Sophie's mother should:

Be patient and supportive: Give Sophie time to express herself, offering encouragement and understanding without interrupting or completing her sentences.

Maintain eye contact and use active listening: Show Sophie that she is genuinely interested in what she says by maintaining eye contact and providing non-verbal cues such as nods or smiles.

Encourage open dialogue: Create a safe and supportive environment for Sophie to express her feelings and thoughts about her stuttering and to discuss any frustrations or concerns she may have.

Offer help when needed: If Sophie is struggling, be prepared to help her in a gentle and non-intrusive way, such as suggesting alternative ways of communicating or asking her if she needs help.

Be a role model of clear and slow speech: When talking with Sophie, set an example using calm and slow speech, which can help her feel more comfortable and make it easier to imitate this speech pattern.

Educate herself about stuttering: Learn about stuttering and the different techniques and therapies available to help Sophie manage her speech. This knowledge will enable her to provide her with evidence-based support and guidance.

8

Story analysis

Summary

In conclusion, Sophie's stuttering is a unique challenge to her daily communication, especially when asking for her favorite cookies at the supermarket. However, with the proper support from her mother and other family members and professional help from speech and language therapists, Sophie can learn to manage her stuttering effectively and communicate more confidently. In addition, practicing relaxation techniques, building her self-esteem, and using alternative forms of communication can significantly help Sophie overcome the barriers associated with her stuttering. It's important that those around her show empathy, understanding, and patience, which can significantly impact Sophie's overall progress and sense of self-esteem.

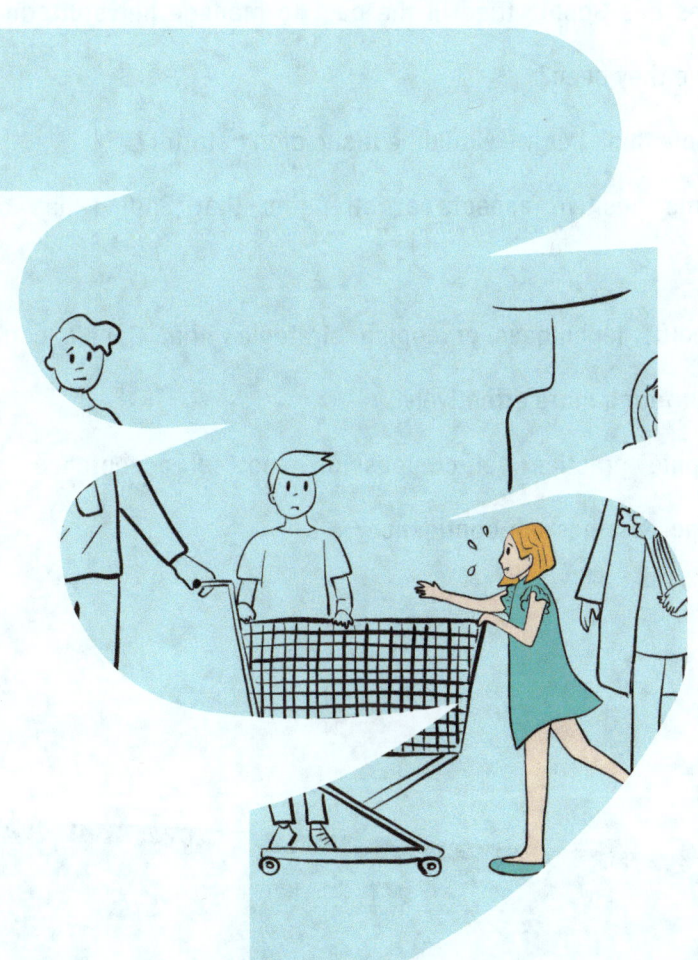

8 Story analysis

Questions...

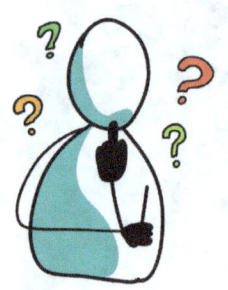

1. On a scale of 1 to 10 (1 = very little, 10 = very much), how much do you think Sophie stutters?

2. How does Sophie feel when she stutters, trying to ask her mother for the cookies?

3. What thoughts go through Sophie's mind when she realizes she is stuttering?

4. Can Sophie identify specific situations or emotions that might trigger her stuttering?

5. How do other people around Sophie react when she stutters, and how does she feel about it?

6. What strategies has Sophie tried in the past to manage her stuttering, and how successful have they been?

7. How does Sophie think her life would be if she didn't stutter?

8. What are some positive aspects or strengths that Sophie has despite her stuttering?

9. Are there specific techniques or coping strategies that Sophie could learn to manage her stuttering more effectively?

10. How can Sophie practice self-compassion and self-acceptance, even when stuttering, to increase her self-confidence?

9 The presentation

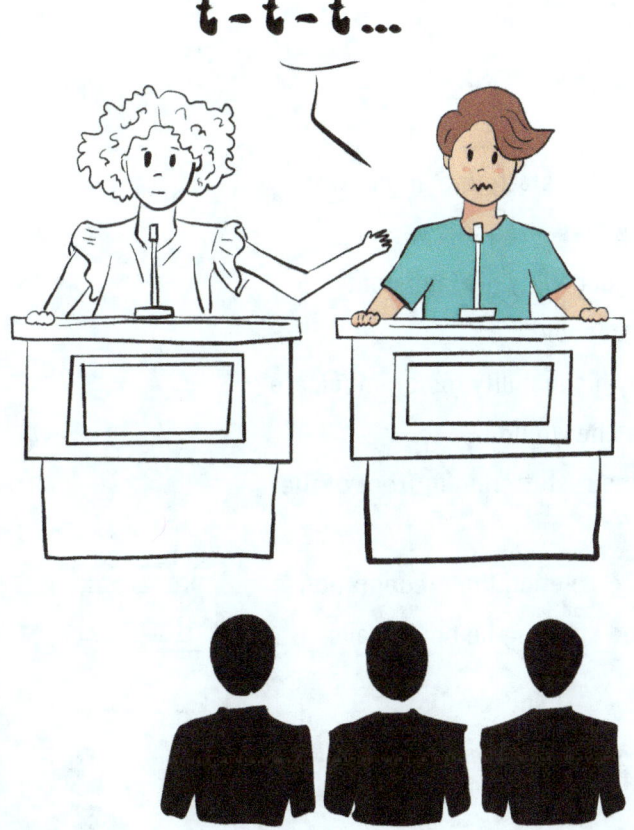

Peter, a teenage student, stands in front of the class to make a presentation with his partner. As he begins to speak, his stuttering becomes more intense, and he feels his anxiety increasing. Despite his best efforts to remain calm, he cannot. Time doesn't seem to pass as he struggles to cope. He is relieved when he finally finishes his speech but knows he could have done better.

Story analysis

From Peter's perspective

A. Thoughts and feelings:

Peter may feel...

- Concerned about his stuttering and how it might affect the presentation.
- Afraid of being judged by his classmates or appearing less capable.
- Disappointed by his inability to communicate as effectively as he would like to.
- Embarrassed about stuttering in front of the class.
- Relieved after completing the presentation but disappointed knowing he could have done better.

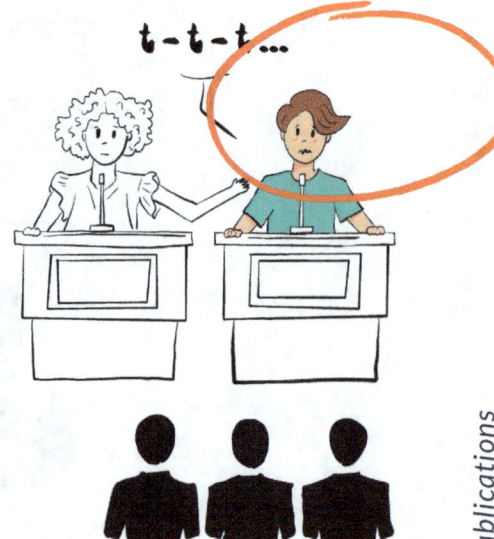

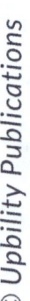

B. Possible actions:

- He could pause and take a few deep breaths to calm down.
- He could rehearse or practice speaking techniques to manage his stuttering in advance.
- He could ask for support from his partner during the presentation.
- He could seek professional help, such as speech therapy, to improve his stuttering in the long term.
- He could explain his stuttering to the class before the presentation to reduce some anxiety.

9 Story analysis

From his partner's perspective

A. Thoughts and feelings:

Peter's presentation partner may feel...

- Empathy for Peter's anxiety and his stuttering during the presentation.
- Concerned that Peter's stuttering may affect the overall presentation.
- Embarrassed or unsure about how to support Peter during the presentation.

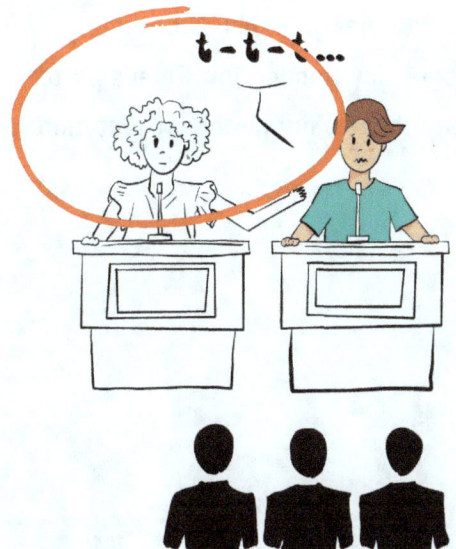

B. Possible actions:

Peter's presentation partner could...

- Step in to help Peter with his presentation when he's struggling.
- Reassure Peter before and after the presentation that they did well together.
- Encourage Peter to seek professional help to manage his stuttering.
- Help Peter practice and prepare more for future presentations.

Story analysis

From the perspective of bystanders

A. Thoughts and feelings:

- Some may feel sympathy for Peter's struggle during the presentation.
- Others may feel uncomfortable or unsure how to react.
- Some classmates may be judgmental or reject Peter due to his stuttering.
- Some may wonder how Peter's partner will react or help during the presentation.

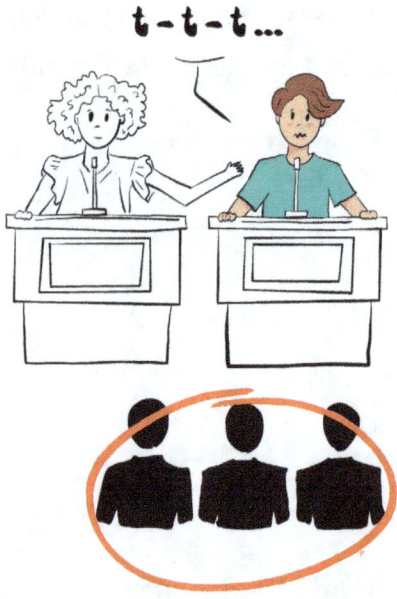

B. Possible actions:

- Providing words of encouragement or support to Peter after the presentation.
- Avoiding negative comments or judgments about Peter's stuttering.
- Being patient and understanding during the presentation.
- Learning more about stuttering to understand Peter's experience better.

Story analysis

Tips for effective communication:

People who stutter should:

Practice relaxation techniques: They can help reduce anxiety and increase concentration during communication.

Talk slowly: Speaking at a slower pace can help manage stuttering and provide greater control over speech.

Use pauses: Strategically introducing pauses during speech can help organize thoughts and manage stuttering more effectively.

Prepare and practice: Rehearsing beforehand can help build confidence and familiarity with the content, facilitating communication during the actual presentation.

Use speech therapy techniques: Working with a speech therapist to learn specific strategies and techniques for managing stuttering can be helpful.

Be open about stuttering: Informing listeners beforehand can relieve some anxiety and create a more supportive audience.

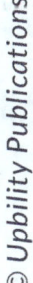

© Upbility Publications

Story analysis

Tips for effective communication:

Peter's presentation partner should:

Actively listen: Pay attention and participate in the conversation, maintaining eye contact and nodding when needed.

Be patient: Give Peter the time he needs to communicate without interrupting him or completing his sentences.

Offer support: If Peter struggles, offer to help or take over part of the presentation to reduce the pressure.

Encourage and offer encouragement and reassurance: Provide positive reinforcement and encouragement to boost Peter's confidence during and after the presentation.

Work with Peter to prepare for the project: Collaborate with Peter to plan and practice the presentation to ensure that both are comfortable with the content and their roles.

Develop clear messages: Ensure that the information presented is well organized and easy to understand, which can help reduce anxiety and stuttering during the presentation.

Story analysis

Summary

In conclusion, effective communication between Peter and his presentation partner involves a combination of preparation, practice, and empathy. By focusing on stuttering management techniques, using relaxation strategies, and developing a supportive environment, Peter can overcome some of the challenges he faces during presentations. Similarly, patience, active listening, and encouragement from his peer can play a key role in creating a successful co-presentation. For both children, incorporating visual aids, clear messaging, and attention to non-verbal communication can further enhance the effectiveness of their communication. Finally, a strong collaborative approach and mutual understanding can help them overcome the challenges of public speaking and deliver a strong presentation.

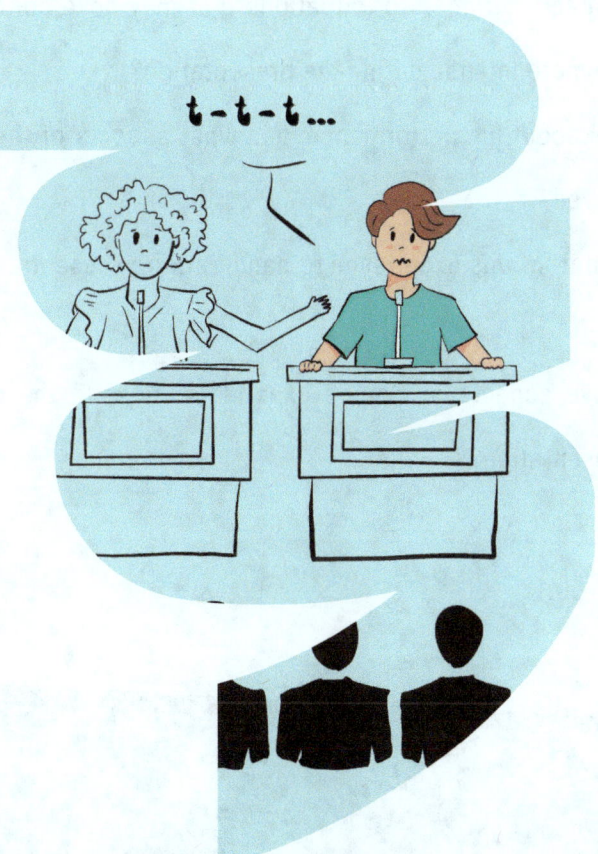

Story analysis

Questions...

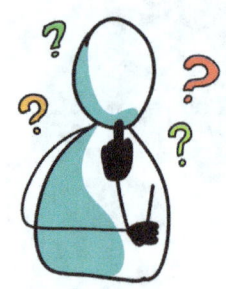

1. On a scale of 1 to 10 (1 = very little, 10 = very much), how much do you think Peter stutters?

2. What are some of the thoughts that go through Peter's mind as he begins to stutter during the presentation?

3. How did Peter's anxiety affect his stuttering during the presentation?

4. What strategies did Peter try to use to remain calm during the presentation, and how successful were they?

5. What could Peter have done differently to better manage his anxiety and stuttering?

6. How did Peter's perception of time during the presentation affect his experience?

7. Can Peter identify specific triggers or situations that may have contributed to his stuttering becoming more intense during the presentation?

8. How does Peter feel about his performance, and what aspects of the presentation could he have improved?

9. What can Peter learn from this experience to handle future presentations or similar situations better?

10. What are the positive aspects of Peter's experience, despite the challenges he faced during the presentation?

10 Rena's book

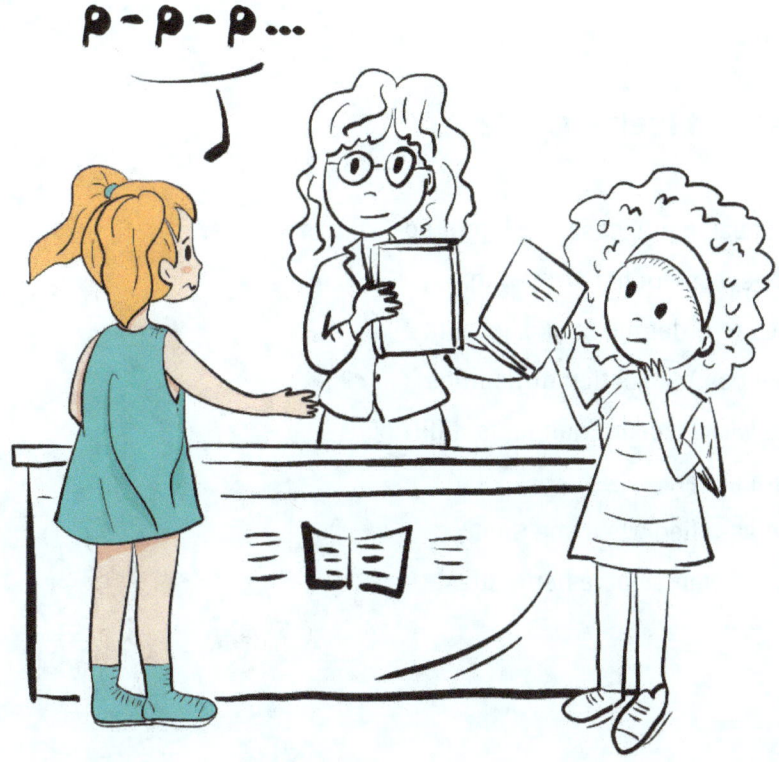

Rena is at the library. "I want a book," she says to the librarian, her voice trembling with anxiety and embarrassment. The clerk looks at Rena, puzzled. "Which book do you want?" she asks. Rena tries to answer, but her stuttering makes it difficult. She tries again, but the librarian still cannot understand what she wants. Frustrated, Rena takes a deep breath and tries again. This time, she speaks slowly and softly. "I want a book about penguins," she says clearly and confidently. The librarian smiles and says: "Oh, I see! Let me get it for you." Rena glows with pride when the librarian hands her the book because even if she struggled at first, she didn't give up and succeeded!

10 Story analysis

From Rena's perspective

A. Thoughts and feelings:

Rena may feel...

- Afraid to speak out in case she might be criticized because of her stuttering.
- Determined to order the book she wants despite her communication difficulties.
- Frustrated when the librarian finds it difficult to understand her.
- Proud and satisfied when she finally manages to communicate her request clearly.

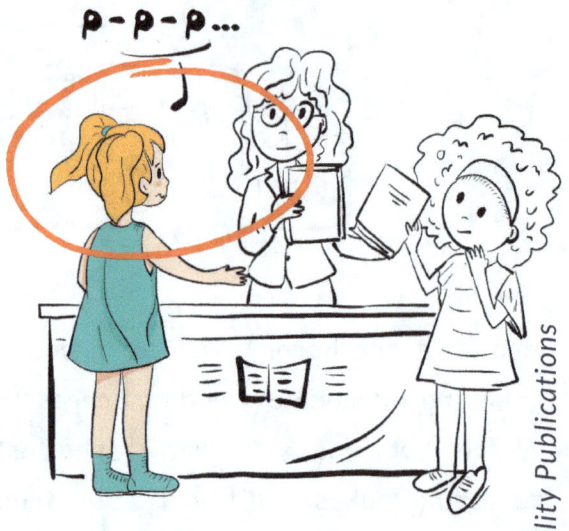

B. Possible actions:

- Rena could have written down her request instead of trying to express it in words.
- She could have practiced her request before reaching out to the librarian.
- Rena could have searched for the book herself or asked a friend for help.

Story analysis

From the librarian's perspective

A. Thoughts and feelings:

The librarian may feel...

- Confused by Rena's request and unsure what she wants.
- Sympathetic to Rena's struggle to communicate her request.
- Satisfied with helping Rena overcome her challenges and achieve her goal.

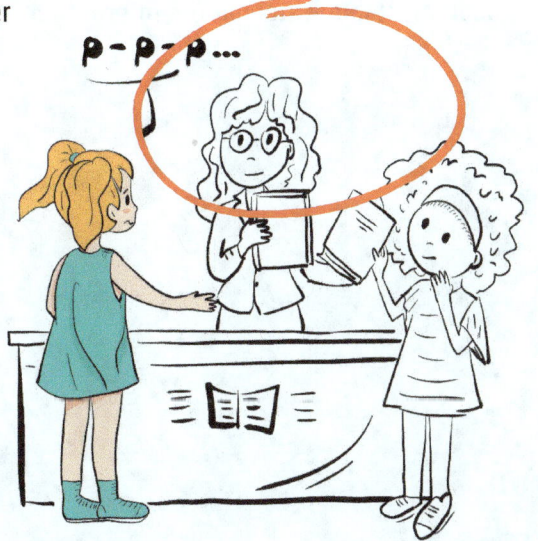

B. Possible actions:

- The librarian could ask Rena to write down her request.
- She could direct her to a computer to look up the book.
- She could wait patiently and respectfully for Rena to complete her sentence.

Story analysis

From the perspective of bystanders

A. Thoughts and feelings:

- Bystanders may feel sympathy for Rena's struggle to communicate her request.
- They may feel impressed or inspired by Rena's determination and persistence.
- Some bystanders may feel embarrassed or uncomfortable watching the interaction.

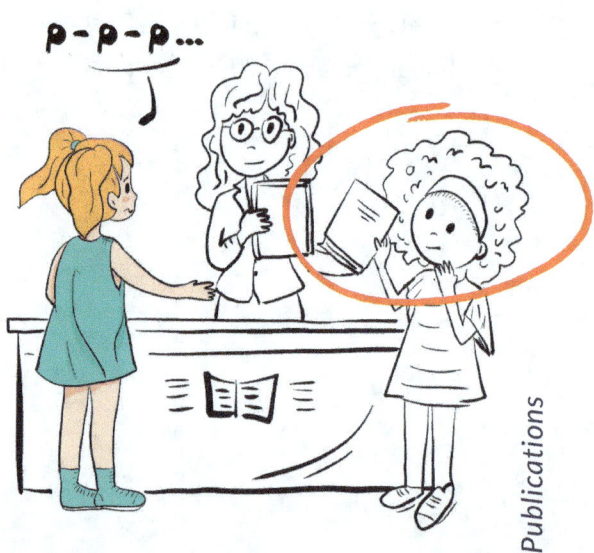

B. Possible actions:

- Bystanders could offer to help Rena by writing her request or helping her find the book.
- They could offer words of encouragement or support to Rena during her struggle.
- They could give space to Rena and the librarian, respecting their privacy during the interaction.

Story analysis

Tips for effective communication:

Rena should:

Relax and breathe: Take a few deep breaths before speaking to calm down and reduce stress, which can only worsen stuttering.

Speak slowly: Speaking slowly and consciously can help her maintain control of her speech and reduce stuttering.

Use short sentences: Breaking long sentences into shorter ones may be easier to express, which can help reduce stuttering.

Practice: Rehearse what she wants to say beforehand to gain confidence and fluency with the words and phrases.

Visualize success: Imagine herself speaking fluently and confidently to boost her self-esteem and create a positive mindset.

Be patient with herself: Remember that stuttering does not reflect her intelligence or abilities. Accept it and not be too hard on herself.

Seek support: Join a support group, go to a speech therapist, or connect with others who stutter to share experiences, advice, and encouragement.

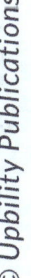

Story analysis

Tips for effective communication:

The librarian should:

Be patient and focused: Give Rena time to express herself and pay close attention to her words to better understand her request.

Encourage non-verbal communication: If Rena finds it difficult to verbally express her request, offer her the opportunity to write it down or use the computer to look up the book.

Maintain eye contact: Maintaining friendly and non-judgmental eye contact can help Rena feel more comfortable and supported.

Avoid interrupting or completing sentences: Allow Rena to complete her thoughts without interruption, as this may cause increased anxiety and worsen stuttering.

Offer reassurance: Offer gentle encouragement and reassurance to help Rena feel comfortable and supported during the interaction.

Create a welcoming environment: Make sure the library is a safe and inviting place for everyone, including those with speech difficulties.

Educate herself: Learn about stuttering and its challenges to better understand and sympathize with people like Rena and be prepared to serve their needs.

Story analysis

Summary

In conclusion, effective communication is essential for Rena and the librarian for their successful interaction. For Rena, finding strategies to manage her stuttering and build self-confidence is crucial. At the same time, the librarian can create an environment of support and understanding to facilitate their interaction. Both parties can benefit from patience, empathy, and a willingness to adapt their communication to meet the needs of the other. By fostering an inviting atmosphere and focusing on clear communication, Rena and the librarian can work together to overcome challenges and ensure a positive experience for all.

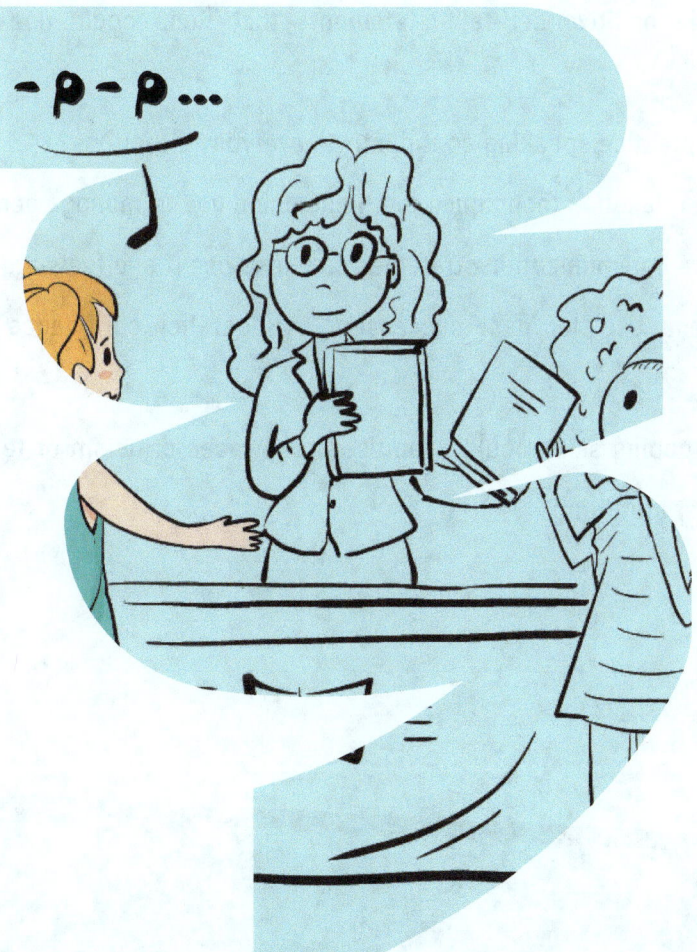

10 Story analysis

Questions...

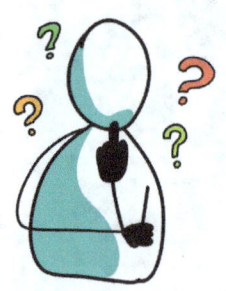

1. On a scale of 1 to 10 (1 = very little, 10 = very much), how much do you think Rena stutters?

2. How did Rena feel when she walked into the library and approached the librarian's desk?

3. What thoughts were going through Rena's mind as she struggled to talk to the librarian?

4. How did Rena overcome her anxiety and embarrassment when she struggled to talk to the librarian?

5. What was the librarian's reaction when Rena spoke slowly and clearly?

6. What are some positive self-talk statements that Rena could use in similar situations?

7. How can Rena practice speaking confidently in everyday situations?

8. What are some relaxation techniques that Rena could use to manage her anxiety?

9. What alternative communication strategies can Rena use if she feels stuck?

10. How might Rena use her past successes to boost her confidence in similar situations?

11. What valuable coping skills could Rena use if she faces criticism or teasing from others about her stuttering?

Bumping into grandmother

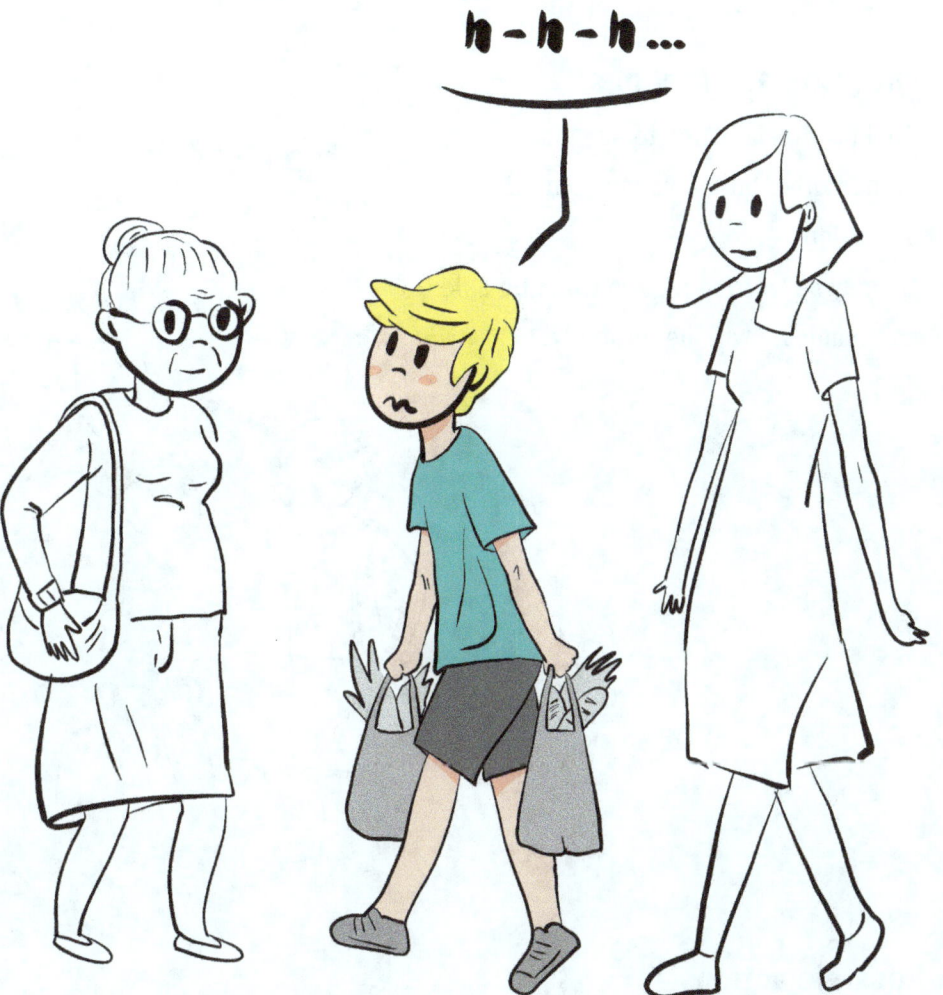

Paul and his mother return home after shopping when they see his grandmother. Paul is excited to see her but also nervous, so he stutters. As they approach each other, Paul's mom notices his discomfort and begins the conversation with her mother. Paul sighs with relief and slowly joins in.

Story analysis

From Paul's perspective

A. Thoughts and feelings:

- Paul may feel excited to see his grandmother but nervous about his stuttering.
- He may be worried that he won't be able to communicate with her properly.

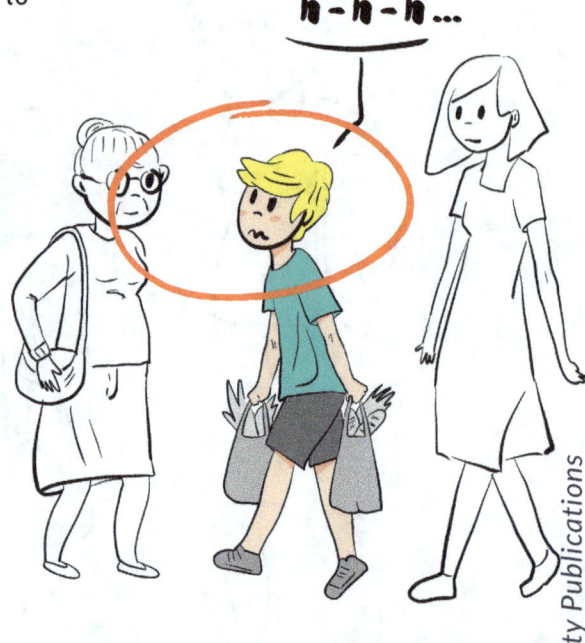

B. Possible actions:

- Paul may avoid speaking and remain silent or speak slowly and carefully to prevent stuttering.
- He may also feel relieved if someone else takes the lead role in the conversation.

Story analysis

From the mother's perspective

A. Thoughts and feelings:

Paul's mother may...

- Notice her son's discomfort and want to support him.
- Empathize with Paul's feelings about his stuttering and try to make the situation more comfortable for him.

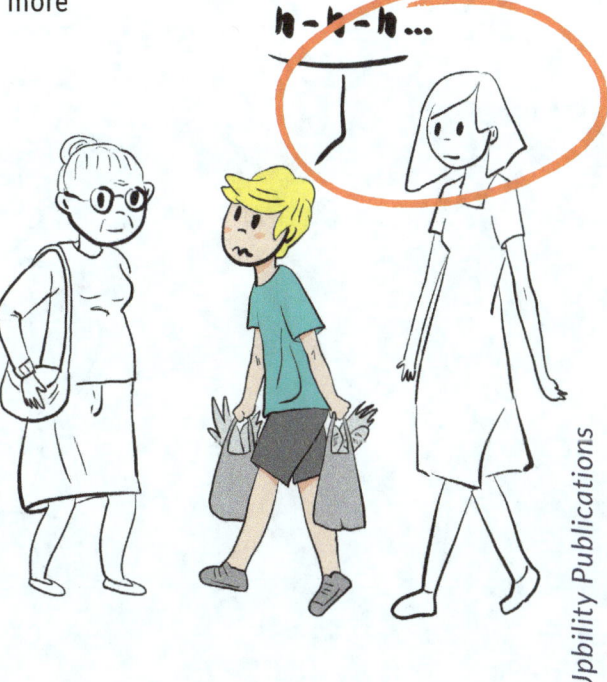

B. Possible actions:

- His mother could intervene and start the conversation to relieve Paul of the pressure.
- She might also encourage him to participate and offer support and reassurance.

Story analysis

From the perspective of bystanders

A. Thoughts and feelings:

- Paul's grandmother may feel happy to see her family and excited to talk to them.
- She may also notice Paul's stuttering and feel empathy toward him.

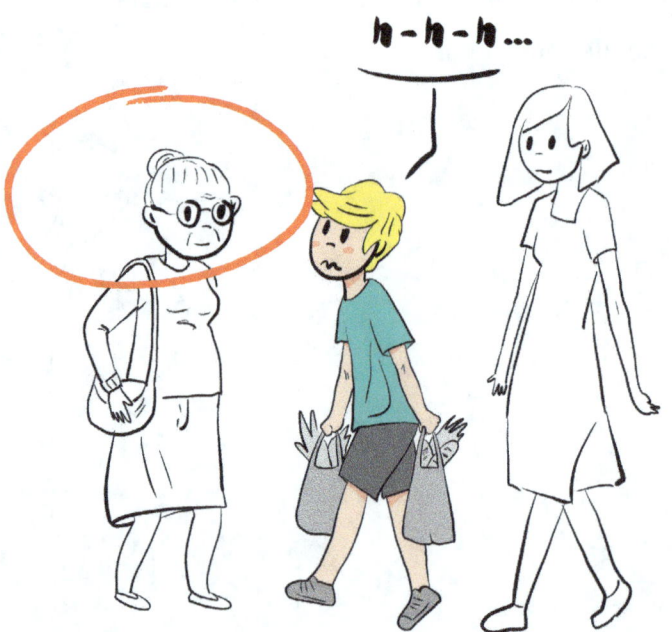

B. Possible actions:

- Paul's grandmother could try to include him in the conversation, even if he stutters, to make him feel comfortable.
- She may offer support and encouragement or ask him questions he can easily answer.

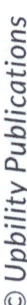

Story analysis

Tips for effective communication:

Speak slowly and clearly: Speaking slowly can help reduce stuttering and make it easier for the listener to understand the message.

Use pauses: Pauses during a conversation can provide an opportunity to gather your thoughts and slow the pace of speech.

Focus on the breath: Taking deep breaths can help relax the body and facilitate comfortable speaking.

Use eye contact: Maintaining eye contact while speaking can help build confidence and connect with the listener.

Be patient and actively listen: Listeners need to be patient and allow time for stuttering speakers to complete their sentences. Active listening can help encourage communication and show support.

Practice and seek help: Practicing communication skills and seeking help from a speech therapist or support group can help people who stutter improve their communication skills.

Avoid interrupting or completing sentences: Interrupting or completing sentences can make the speaker feel incompetent. Allowing the speaker to complete their sentences can help build confidence and reduce stuttering.

Stay positive: Stuttering can be frustrating, but keeping a positive attitude and focusing on strengths and successes can help build confidence and improve communication skills.

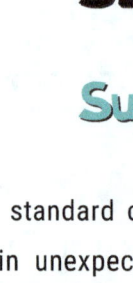

Story analysis

Summary

Paul's stuttering is a standard communication challenge many people face and can be particularly difficult in unexpected meetings or other social gatherings. However, as shown in the incident with his grandmother, there are several ways to manage stuttering and communicate effectively. With patience, practice, and support, people like Paul can improve their communication skills and feel more confident in social situations. Understanding and support from family members and friends, such as Paul's mother and grandmother, can make a significant difference and help people with stuttering feel more comfortable and valued in their interactions.

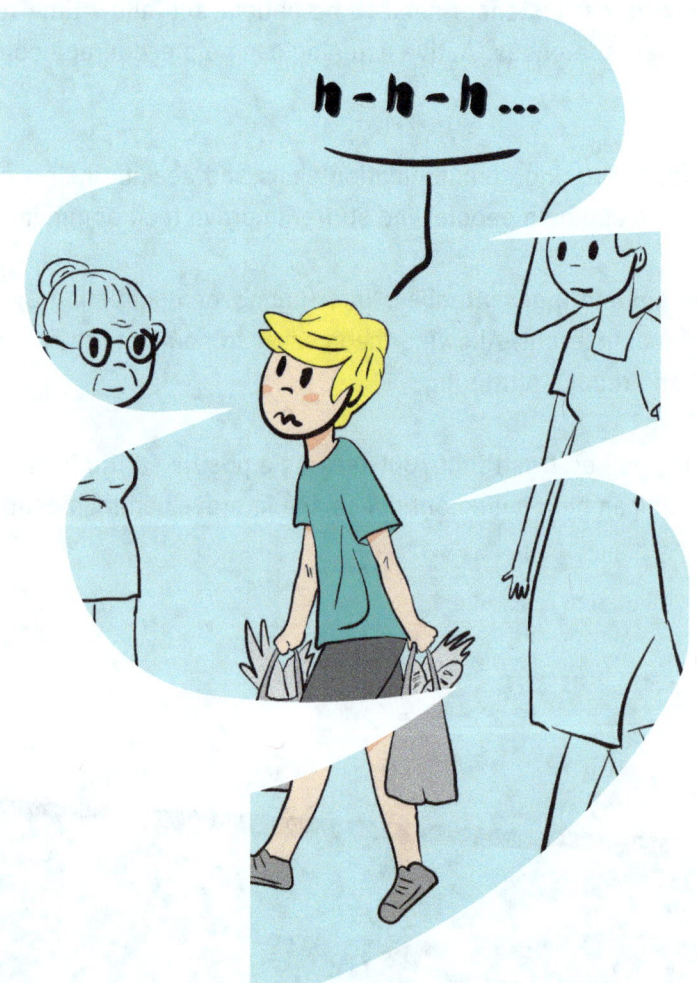

Story analysis

Questions...

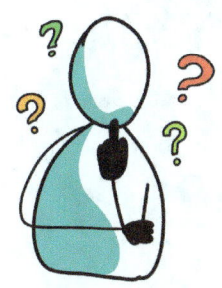

1. On a scale of 1 to 10 (1=slightly, 10=very much), how much do you think Paul stutters?

2. How do you think Paul feels when he starts to stutter?

3. What thoughts go through Paul's mind as he waits to talk to his grandmother?

4. How does Paul's mother's intervention help him in this situation?

5. How might Paul's feelings about his stuttering affect his interaction with his grandmother?

6. What strategies could Paul use to feel more comfortable talking to his grandmother?

7. How could Paul's mother help him become more confident when talking with his grandmother despite his stuttering?

8. Can you identify the positive aspects of Paul's interaction with his grandmother?

9. How might Paul's stuttering change as he gets older and gains more experience in social situations?

10. How would you feel if you were in Paul's shoes, and what would you do differently in this story?

 # Remaining silent

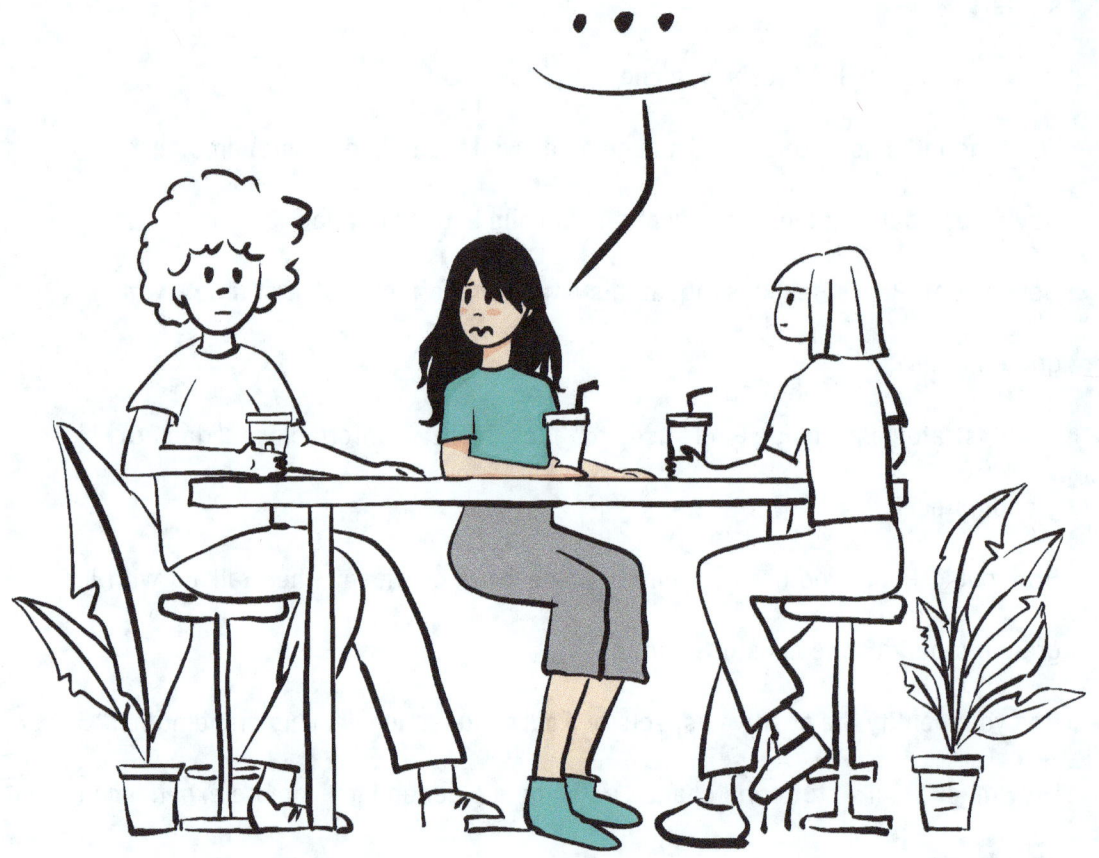

Rhea and her friends are in a café. While her friends are talking, Rhea remains silent. She is afraid of stuttering and feels anxious when someone speaks to her. Rhea doesn't want to embarrass herself in front of her friends, so she remains silent, hoping no one will notice. Rhea wishes she were more confident and could speak without hesitating, but the fear of stuttering keeps holding her back.

Story analysis

From Rhea's perspective

A. Thoughts and feelings:

Rhea may feel...

- Anxious, frustrated, and afraid of stuttering.
- Worried about how her friends would react if she stuttered or how embarrassing it would be for her.
- Disappointed in herself for not being able to speak confidently and wished she could overcome her fear.

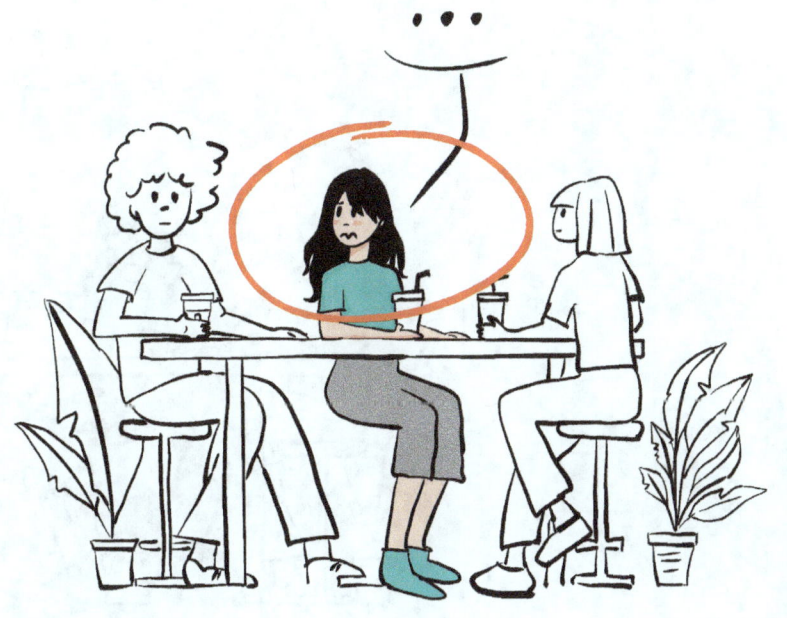

B. Possible actions:

- Rhea may remain silent, hoping no one will notice her anxiety.
- Alternatively, she could participate in the conversation by speaking slowly or using non-verbal cues such as nods or facial expressions.
- Rhea could also consider sharing her feelings and fear of stuttering with a close friend, seeking support and understanding.

12 Story analysis

From Rhea's friend's perspective

A. Thoughts and feelings:

Rhea's friend may...

- Feel concerned about seeing Rhea so silent.
- Be wondering if she's upset or not interested in the conversation.
- Be confused about Rhea's behavior, unaware of her fear of stuttering.

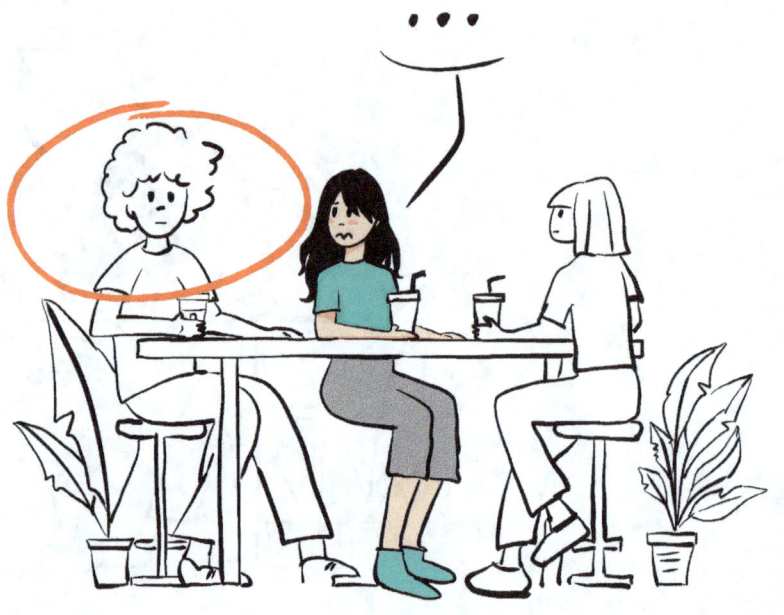

B. Possible actions:

- Rhea's friend can try to include her in the conversation by asking her questions or sharing stories about her.
- She could also ask Rhea privately if everything is okay or if there is anything she can do to help. If Rhea shares her fear, her friend can offer support, encouragement, or advice to help her feel more comfortable.

Story analysis

From the perspective of bystanders

A. Thoughts and feelings:

- Bystanders may not notice Rhea's silence or anxiety, being occupied with their conversations.
- They may feel curious or confused about why Rhea isn't participating.

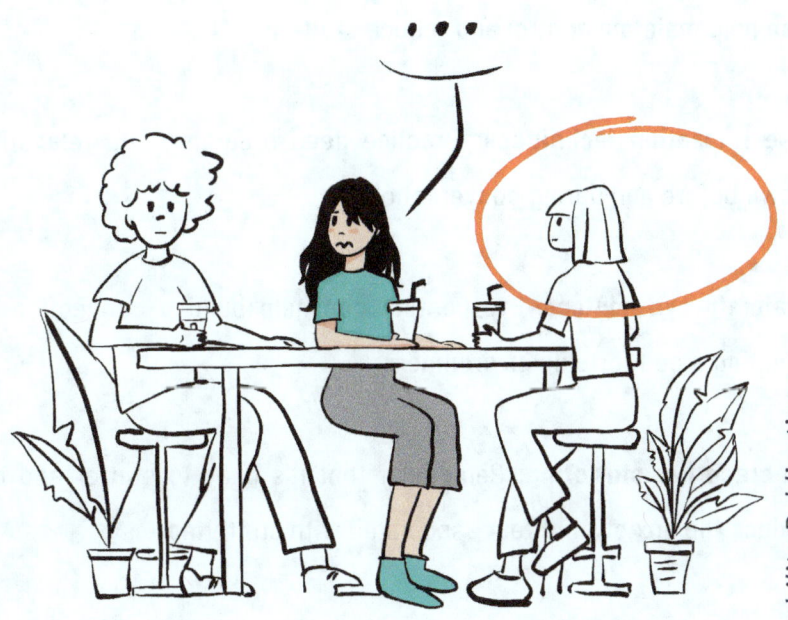

© Upbility Publications

B. Possible actions:

Bystanders may choose to respect her privacy and not interfere. Alternatively, they could include Rhea in the conversation or offer her a friendly smile, helping her feel more comfortable. However, it's important that bystanders are sensitive to Rhea's feelings and do not make her the center of attention, which may make her feel more uncomfortable.

Story analysis

Tips for effective communication:

Rhea should:

Prepare and practice: Before entering a conversation, consider preparing and practicing what she wants to say. This will help her reduce anxiety and gain confidence in speaking.

Speak slowly: Take time while speaking, and not feel pressured to rush. Speaking slowly can help maintain control and reduce stuttering.

Use relaxation techniques: Practice deep breathing and relaxation techniques to calm down before and during conversations.

Maintain eye contact: Eye contact can help build a connection with the other person, creating a comfortable environment.

Embrace her stuttering: Remember that it's okay to stutter and be open. This can help reduce the anxiety and fear associated with stuttering.

Seek professional help: Consider seeing a speech and language therapist or joining a support group to learn strategies for managing stuttering and building confidence in communication.

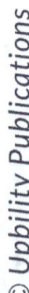

12 Story analysis

Tips for effective communication:

Rhea's friend should:

Be patient: Give Rhea time to express herself without interrupting or completing her sentences. This shows respect and understanding.

Maintain eye contact: Eye contact helps Rhea feel more comfortable and shows that she is genuinely interested in what she is saying.

Avoid criticism: Be empathetic and supportive, avoiding any criticism or negative reaction to Rhea's stuttering.

Encourage participation: Include Rhea in conversations by asking open-ended questions or sharing relevant stories. This can help her feel more comfortable and confident when participating.

Provide positive reinforcement: Reinforce Rhea's contribution to the discussion by focusing on her message rather than her speech.

Learn about stuttering: Educate about stuttering and its challenges to better understand and support Rhea. This can also help her become a more effective and empathetic listener.

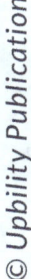

Story analysis

Summary

In conclusion, the story of Rhea in the café shows the challenges faced by people who stutter and the importance of empathy and understanding from their peers. Rhea's fear of stuttering and the anxiety she experiences in social situations such as this can be a significant obstacle in her daily life. However, with the support and encouragement of her friends, Rhea can begin to overcome her fears and gain confidence in her communication skills. By practicing effective communication strategies and seeking professional help, Rhea can learn to manage her stuttering and participate confidently in social situations. In addition, her friends can play a key role in creating a comfortable and welcoming environment, allowing Rhea to express herself more openly and without criticism. Rhea's story serves as a reminder that stuttering should not define a person's worth and that empathy, patience, and understanding are essential to fostering positive and supportive relationships.

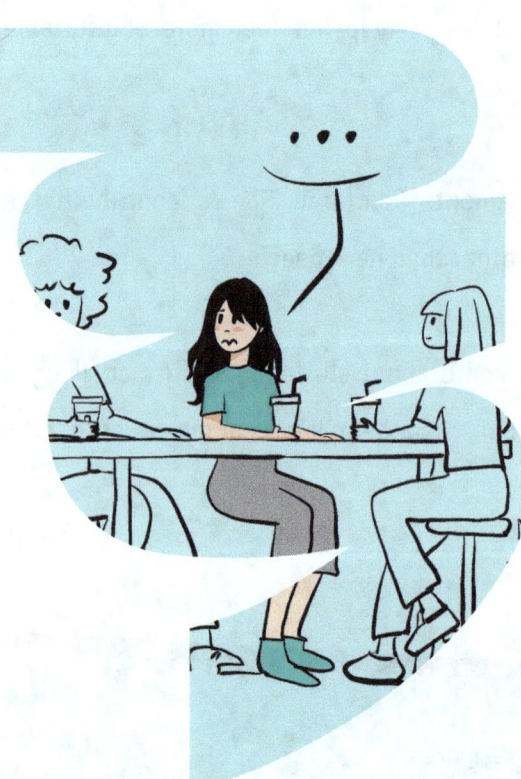

Story analysis

Questions...

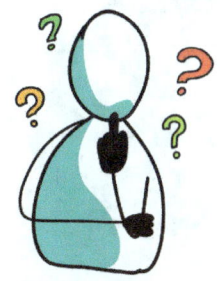

1. On a scale of 1 to 10 (1 = very little, 10 = very much), how much do you think Rhea stutters?

2. How does Rhea feel when she stutters?

3. What thoughts go through Rhea's mind when she thinks about talking to her friends?

4. What is Rhea's biggest fear about stuttering in front of her friends?

5. Can Rhea think of a time when she stuttered, but it didn't turn out as badly as she thought?

6. How do Rhea's friends react when she stutters? Do they support her or make fun of her?

7. What positive qualities Rhea has that are unrelated to her stuttering?

8. How would Rhea's life be different if she was fearless of stuttering?

9. What steps can Rhea take to feel more comfortable and confident when she speaks?

10. How can Rhea challenge her negative thoughts about stuttering and replace them with more realistic and positive ones?

13 On a date

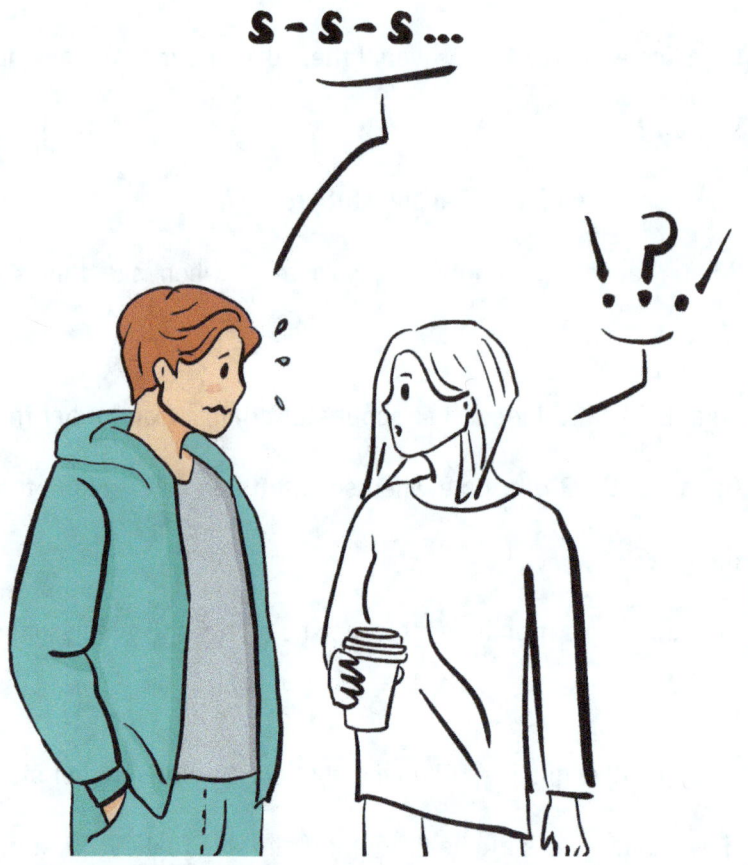

Luke's heart pounds as he approaches his classmate, Sarah, after class. He tries to ask her out on a date, but his stutter makes it difficult to express his feelings. His words stumble, and he feels awkward. Sarah smiles and waits patiently for him to finish. Finally, Luke manages to ask her out, and Sarah agrees, impressed by his bravery. Luke's heart soars as he walks away, grateful for Sarah's understanding and joyful for their upcoming date.

Story analysis

From Luke's perspective

A. Thoughts and feelings:

Luke may feel...

- Nervous and anxious as he approaches Sarah to ask her out on a date.
- Worried about her reaction and his ability to effectively communicate his feelings due to his stuttering.
- Embarrassed and lacking confidence as he speaks.
- A mixture of relief, happiness, and gratitude for Sarah's patience and understanding after she agreed to the date.

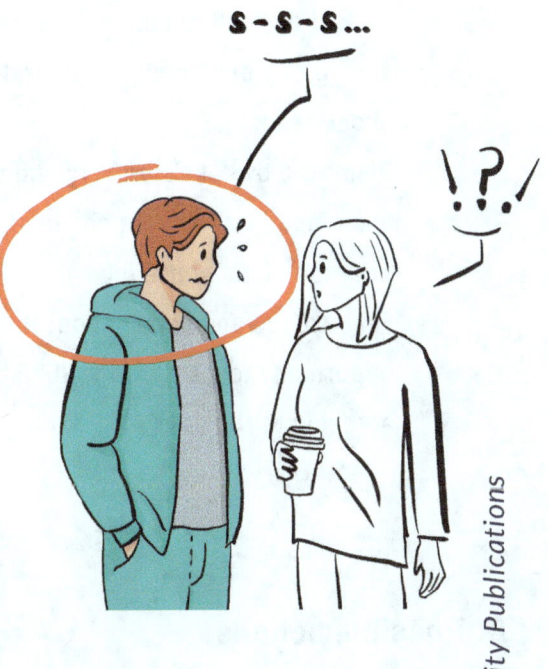

B. Possible actions:

Luke could:

- Take a deep breath before approaching Sarah to calm down.
- Try to speak slowly and softly to minimize his stuttering.
- Rehearse in his mind what he wants to say before he speaks.
- Express gratitude for Sarah's patience.
- Smile and thank her for her reaction.

 **Story analysis**

From Sarah's perspective

A. Thoughts and feelings:

Sarah may...

- Be curious about what Luke wants to say as he approaches her.
- Initially feel embarrassed or worried as he finds it difficult to communicate his feelings, she quickly becomes patient and understanding.
- Be moved by Luke's bravery and persistence, and empathize with the challenges he faces because of his stuttering.
- Feel excited and happy about the opportunity to get to know Luke better after agreeing to the date.

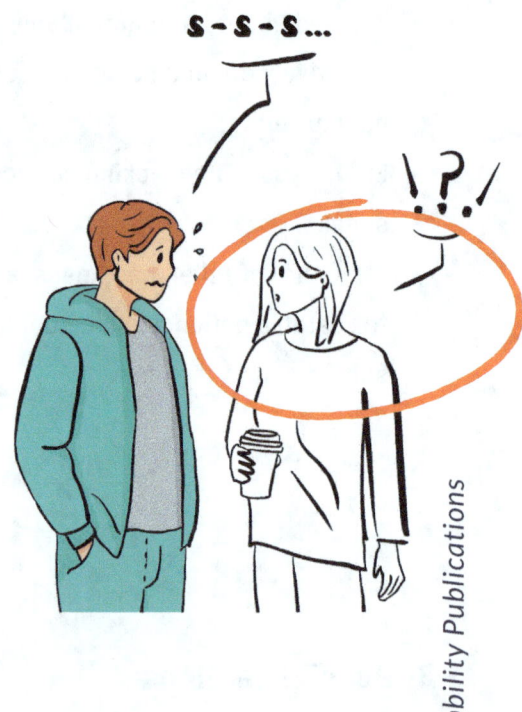

B. Possible actions:

Sarah could:

- Listen carefully to Luke and maintain eye contact.
- Smile at him and offer encouragement if he is struggling with his stuttering.
- Wait patiently for him to finish talking without interrupting or completing his sentences.
- Express understanding and empathy for his stuttering.
- Refrain from commenting on his speech, but focus on the meaning of his words.

13 Story analysis

Tips for effective communication:

Luke should:

Stay relaxed: Focus on maintaining a calm attitude, taking deep breaths, and not getting upset if stuttering occurs.

Practice: Rehearse what he needs to say before the conversation to gain confidence and become comfortable with the words.

Speak slowly: Try speaking slower, which can help control stuttering and allow for more time to form his words.

Use pauses: Pause between words or sentences to gather his thoughts and regain speech control.

Maintain eye contact: Eye contact shows confidence and helps build a connection with the listener.

Be patient: Give the listener time to process the information and avoid getting frustrated if there is a need to repeat something.

© Upbility Publications

Story analysis

Tips for effective communication:

Sarah should:

Be patient: Give Luke enough time to express his thoughts without interrupting or completing his sentences.

Maintain eye contact: Eye contact shows she cares and helps create a comfortable environment for the speaker.

Offer encouragement: Use physical expressions, such as smiles or nods, to encourage Luke to continue speaking.

Show empathy: Show understanding and support for Luke's challenges, making it clear that stuttering does not affect the value of his message.

Actively listen: Focus on the content of the message rather than the stuttering to ensure proper understanding and meaningful engagement.

Ask for clarification: If necessary, politely and respectfully ask Luke to clarify any unclear points due to his stuttering while affirming her appreciation for his efforts to communicate.

By following these tips, Luke and Sarah can work together to create a more effective and comfortable communication experience.

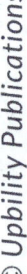

Story analysis

Summary

As Luke and Sarah embarked on their new journey together, they discovered the true power of understanding, patience, and empathy. Despite the challenges presented by Luke's stuttering, their relationship strengthened as they learned to communicate effectively and appreciate each other's unique qualities. Over time, Luke's confidence grew, and his stuttering gradually became a less significant aspect of their conversations. Sarah's constant support and attention allowed her to see beyond his speech difficulty, recognizing the depth and intelligence beneath. Together, they developed a strong bond based on mutual respect and acceptance, proving that genuine connection overcomes speech limitations and that love can blossom despite difficulties.

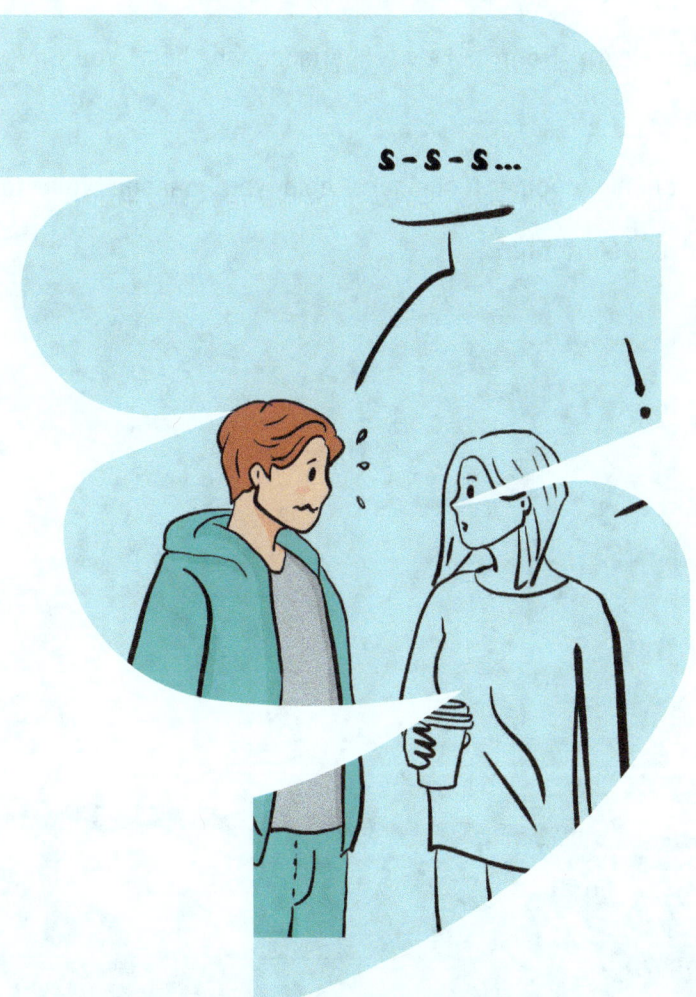

13 Story analysis

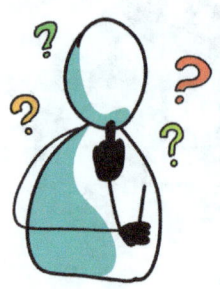

Questions...

1. On a scale of 1 to 10 (1 = very little, 10 = very much), how much do you think Luke stutters?

2. How do you think Luke felt when he approached Sarah to ask her out on a date?

3. What are some positive qualities Luke showed in this story?

4. Can you identify any negative thoughts Luke may have had during this interaction?

5. How did Sarah's reaction to his stuttering make him feel?

6. How could Luke have redefined his thoughts about his stuttering in this situation?

7. How would you handle a similar situation if you were in Luke's position?

8. How do you think Sarah might feel during this interaction?

9. What could you learn from Luke's experience to help you in your social interactions?

10. How might practicing coping techniques help you manage your feelings and thoughts about your stuttering?

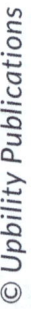

14 Tree-planting

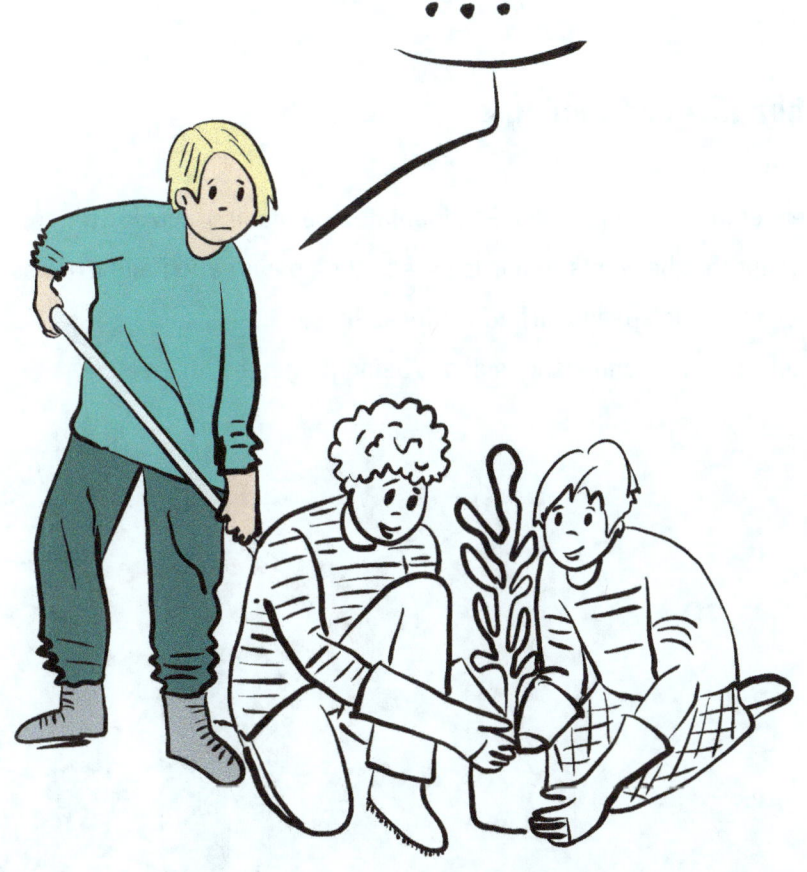

Nick's heart pounds as he digs beside his classmates, trying to follow their conversation. He desperately wants to participate, but the words won't come out of his mouth due to his stuttering. He feels frustrated and embarrassed, wondering if his classmates notice it. Nick wishes he could explain his speech problem but fears being judged. Instead, he remains silent, focusing on planting his tree and hoping for a better tomorrow.

14 Story analysis

From Nick's perspective

A. Thoughts and feelings:

Nick may...

- Feel embarrassed, nervous, and isolated because of his stuttering.
- Accept that he wants to participate in the conversation and express his ideas, but his speech difficulty blocks him.
- Feel frustrated and anxious about being judged by his peers.

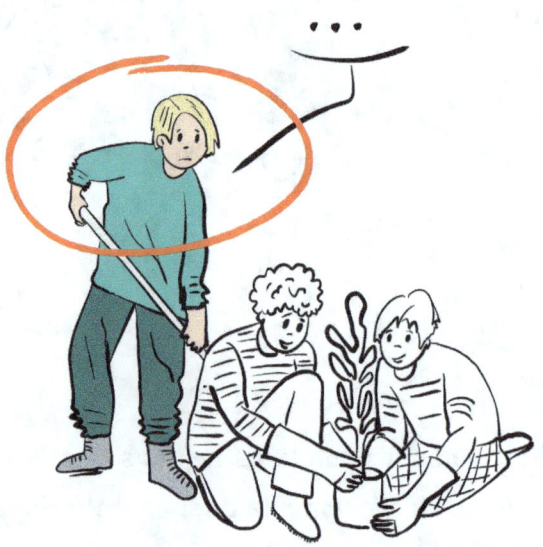

B. Possible actions:

- Nick could remain silent and focus on planting the tree.
- Alternatively, he could try a different way to participate in the conversation, such as body language.
- He could also seek support from a teacher or trusted friend to help him overcome his fear of being criticized and find the courage to participate.

Story analysis

From the classmate's perspective

A. Thoughts and feelings:

Nick's classmate may feel...

- Curious about why Nick doesn't participate in the conversation. He may or may not be aware of his stuttering.

- Anxious or insecure about how to approach the situation. If he knows Nick's speech disorder, he may feel sympathetic or unsure how to help.

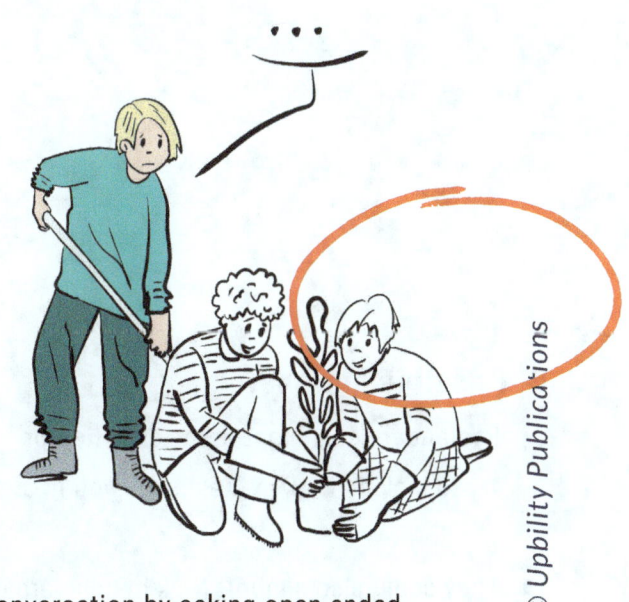

B. Possible actions:

- His classmate could include Nick in the conversation by asking open-ended questions or addressing him in a gentle and supportive way.

- He could also try to engage with Nick in a non-verbal way, such as asking for his help with homework or asking for his opinion through gestures. If classmates know Nick's stuttering, they can be patient and understanding when he speaks up.

Story analysis

From the perspective of bystanders

A. Thoughts and feelings:

- The other children may be curious about Nick's lack of participation or unaware of his struggle.

- They might have mixed feelings about the situation, like empathy, confusion, and indifference.

- Some may be aware of Nick's stuttering and feel anxious or uncertain about how to help.

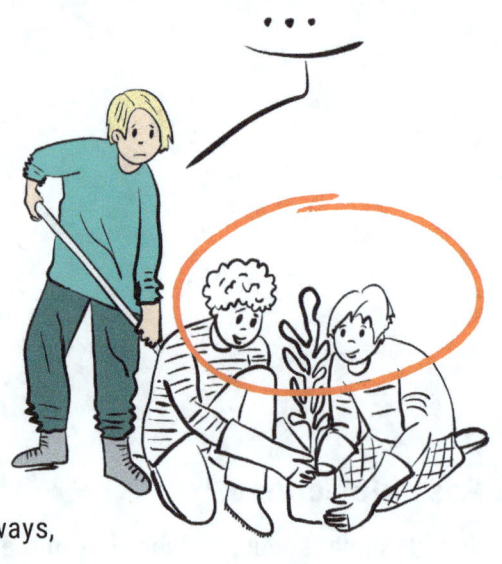

B. Possible actions:

- Bystanders could ignore the situation or try to include Nick in the discussion in a gentle way.

- They could also support Nick in non-verbal ways, such as offering a smile or an encouraging nod.

- If they know his speech difficulty, they can show patience and understanding when he tries to speak, creating a more comfortable environment for his participation.

14 Story analysis

Tips for effective communication:

- **Practice breathing exercises:** Focusing on deep, controlled breathing can help you remain calm and reduce disfluency. Before speaking, take a few deep breaths to concentrate and prepare for the conversation.

- **Take your time:** Speak slowly and gently, giving yourself time to think about what you want to say. This can help relieve the pressure to speak quickly and reduce the frequency of blocks or repetitions.

- **Use alternative methods of communication:** If you find it difficult to speak, consider using non-verbal forms of communication, such as writing or gestures, to communicate your thoughts and ideas.

- **Develop a personal "safe phrase":** Choose a phrase or word you can confidently and without stuttering. Use it to ease into a conversation, providing yourself with a sense of control and confidence.

- **Break the words into smaller parts:** If you struggle with certain words, try breaking them into smaller syllables or sounds. This can help you pronounce them more easily and reduce the chance of blocking.

- **Focus on the message:** Focus on the content of your message rather than your stuttering. This change of focus can help reduce anxiety and improve speech flow.

- **Create a support system:** Surround yourself with people who understand and support your speech disorder. Having a solid support system can help relieve the pressure to speak perfectly and allow you to communicate more effectively.

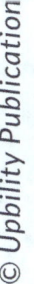

Story analysis

Tips for effective communication:

- **Seek professional help:** Consider working with a speech and language therapist who can provide personalized guidance and strategies to manage your stuttering and improve your communication skills.

- **Practice self-compassion:** Recognize that stuttering is not a personal failure but a challenge that you can work through. Be kind to yourself and acknowledge your progress, whether slow or gradual.

- **Gradual exposure:** Challenge yourself to engage in conversations, starting with low-pressure situations and gradually moving to more challenging contexts. This can help you gain confidence in your communication skills and reduce your fear of stuttering in social situations.

Story analysis

Summary

As time passed, Nick learned to accept and cope with his stuttering, gradually embracing it as part of himself. He discovered that his true friends and supportive classmates valued him for his ideas and character, not his fluency. With the guidance of a speech therapist, he developed strategies to communicate more effectively, even when he stuttered. Nick's newfound confidence allowed him to face his fears and engage in conversations, discovering that the more he practiced, the less scary it became. By focusing on the content of his message rather than his stuttering, Nick found that he could connect with others and make a meaningful impact. Although the journey was not always easy, Nick's persistence and determination to overcome his fear of stuttering ultimately led him to a more fulfilling life where he could embrace his true self and enjoy connecting with those close to him.

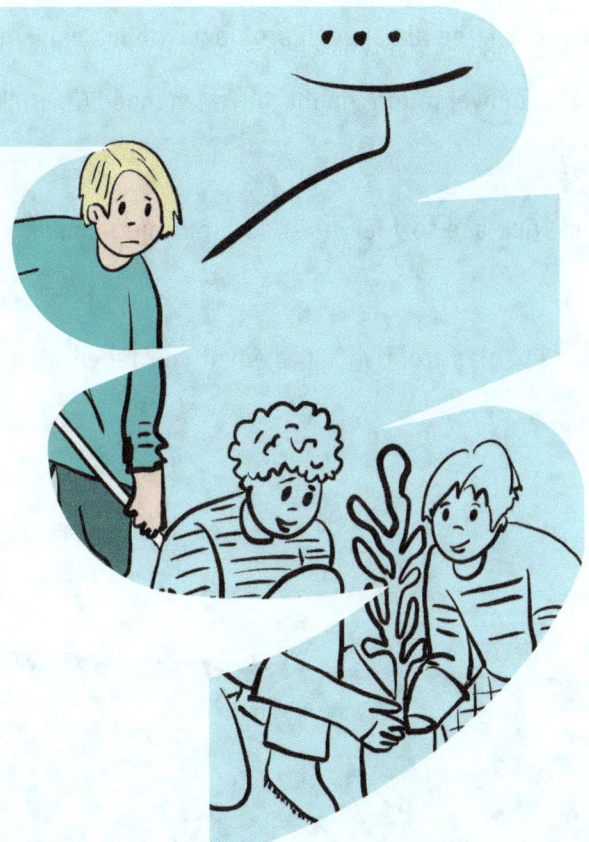

Story analysis

Questions...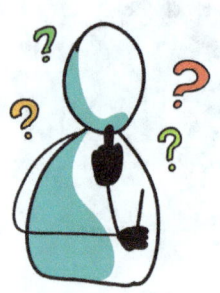

1. On a scale of 1 to 10 (1 = very little, 10 = very much), how much do you think Nick stutters?

2. What thoughts go through Nick's mind when he wants to participate in the conversation but hesitates because of his stuttering?

3. What specific fears does Nick have about whether others will judge him because of his stuttering?

4. How would Nick's classmates react if he stuttered while talking to them?

5. Can you think of any positive characteristics or advantages Nick has that might not relate to his stuttering?

6. How could Nick deal with his frustration and embarrassment about his stuttering in this situation?

7. How might Nick feel if he shared his speech problem with his classmates?

8. How do you think the conversation might have changed if Nick participated, despite his stuttering?

9. What strategies could Nick use to feel more comfortable speaking in front of his classmates?

10. Can you think of any examples from your life when you faced a similar situation? How did you deal with it?

15 Sweet moments

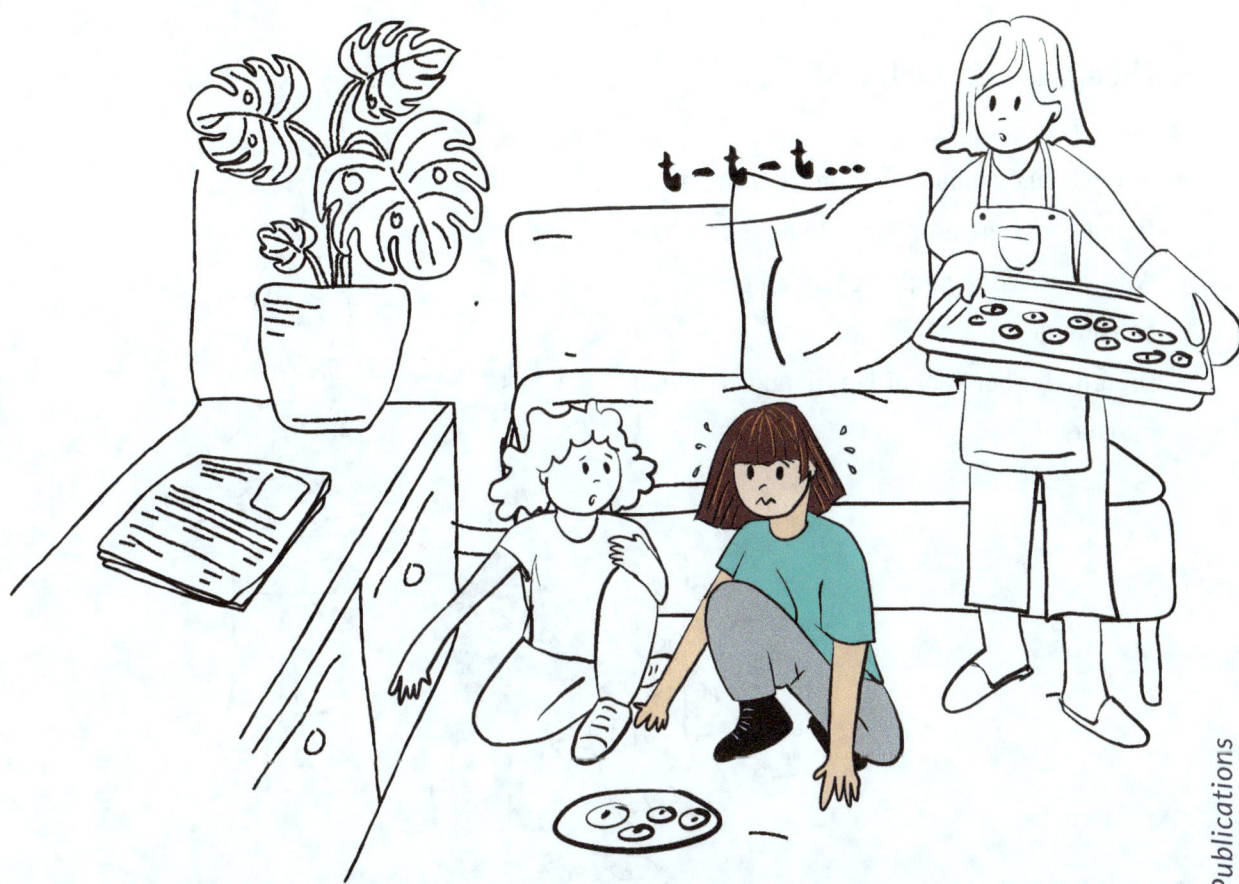

Mary is in her room with a friend. Looking at the plate of freshly baked cookies, she feels nervous and embarrassed. Her friend reaches out to take one, and Mary tries to speak, but her words are stuck in her throat. Her friend looks confused. She doesn't understand what's going on. Mary's mom kindly explains that Mary sometimes has trouble speaking fluently. They enjoy the cookies together, with her friend offering encouragement and support. Mary feels grateful for her supportive friend and loving mother.

Story analysis

From Mary's perspective

A. Thoughts and feelings:

Mary may feel...

- Nervous and embarrassed in front of her friend about the problem with her speech.
- Worried that she might be judged or considered different.
- Grateful for her supportive friend and loving mother.

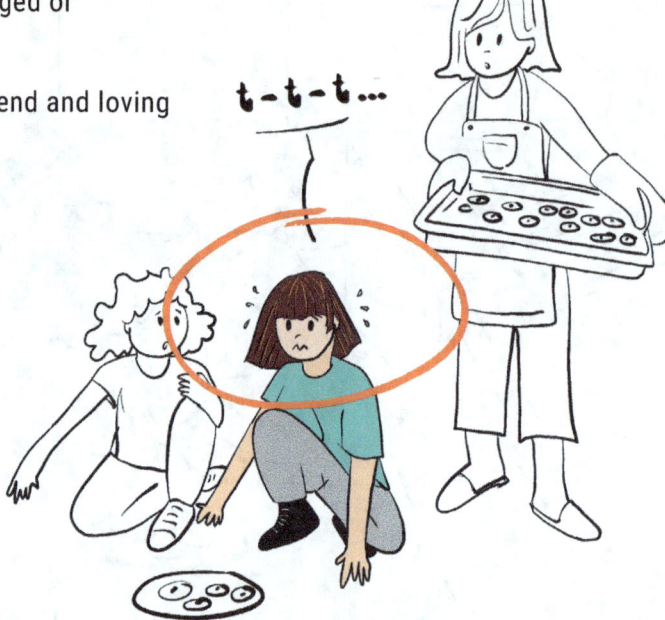

B. Possible actions:

Mary could...

- Try to communicate non-verbally with her friend to express her feelings.
- Try to overcome her speech problem and talk, even if it is difficult.
- Use speech therapy practices to improve her fluency.
- Open up to her friend about her disfluency.
- Thank her friend and her mother for their support and understanding.

15 Story analysis

From the mother's perspective

A. Thoughts and feelings:

Mary's mother may...

- Feel concerned and understanding for her daughter.
- Be thinking of ways to support and help Mary with her speech disorder.
- Appreciate her daughter's friend's understanding and support.

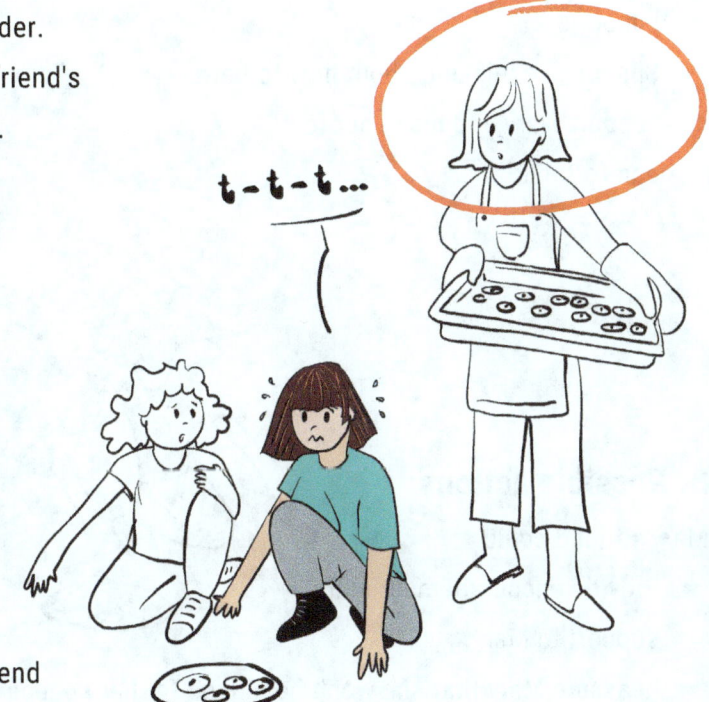

B. Possible actions:

Mary's mother could:

- Gently explain to Mary's friend her speech problem.
- Offer support and encouragement to Mary.
- Encourage her to seek help.
- Help her practice her speech in a comfortable and supportive environment.

Story analysis

From the perspective of bystanders

A. Thoughts and feelings:

- Mary's friend may initially feel confused, not understanding the situation. Once Mary's mother explains the situation, her friend may feel empathy for Mary and want to offer support.
- She may be thinking about how to better support Mary and make her feel comfortable.

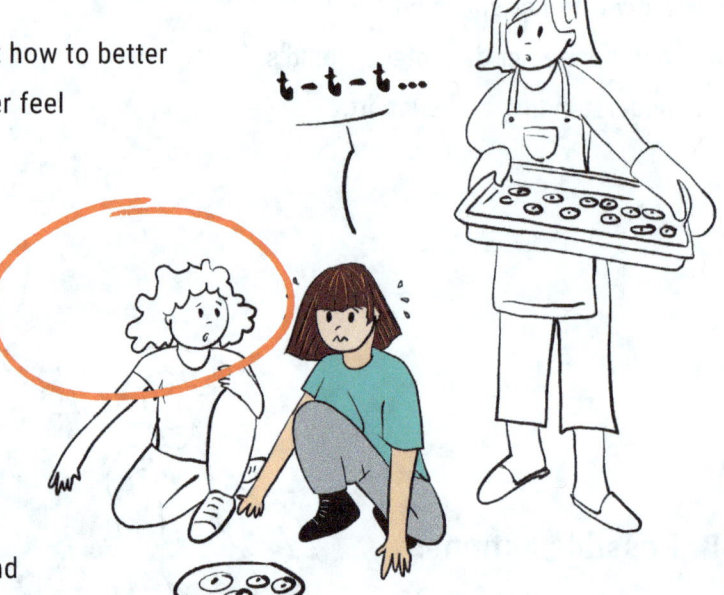

B. Possible actions:

Mary's friend could:

- Provide encouragement and support to Mary.
- Reassure Mary that she won't be judged for her speech disorder.
- Ask Mary or her mother how she can help or support Mary.
- Engage in activities that help Mary feel more comfortable such as non-verbal games.
- Continue to be a supportive friend and maintain open communication.

15 Story analysis

Tips for effective communication:

Mary should:

Practice relaxation techniques: Learn deep breathing exercises and practice them to manage stress and remain calm during conversations.

Speak slowly: Take her time while speaking and not rush to complete her sentences. This can help reduce stuttering and allow smoother speech.

Use pauses: Make pauses in her speech to help her control her communication.

Work with a speech and language therapist: A speech and language therapist can provide guidance and techniques that suit her needs and help manage her stuttering.

Prepare in advance: If she knows she will speak on a particular topic, practice what she wants to say to feel more confident and prepared.

Focus on the message: Remember that the most important aspect of communication is the message being communicated. Try to ignore her stutter as much as possible.

Build confidence: Engage in activities that help her build confidence and self-esteem, which can positively impact her communication skills.

15 Story analysis

Tips for effective communication:

Mary's mother and friend should:

Be patient: Give Mary time to express herself without interrupting or completing her sentences.

Maintain eye contact: Show that you are actively listening and participating in the conversation by maintaining eye contact.

Avoid completing sentences: Resist the urge to complete Mary's sentences, which may discourage and undermine her confidence.

Encourage open communication: Create a supportive environment where Mary feels comfortable talking about her stuttering and any related concerns.

Don't focus on the stuttering: Focus on what Mary says rather than the way she says it.

Offer support: If Mary is working with a speech and language therapist or practicing techniques to manage her stuttering, offer encouragement and support.

Encourage participation: Include Mary in conversations and social situations to help her gain confidence and practice her communication skills.

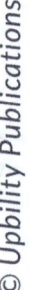

Story analysis

Summary

In summary, effective communication plays a key role in building and maintaining relationships for both Mary and her loved ones. By practicing techniques that work for her, Mary can control her stuttering and improve her communication skills. At the same time, her loved ones can create a supportive environment by being patient, maintaining eye contact, and focusing on the content of the conversation. Through these efforts, Mary can gain confidence in her communication skills and become more comfortable in social situations. By promoting understanding, empathy, and open communication, Mary and her loved ones can improve their relationships and create a positive and supportive environment.

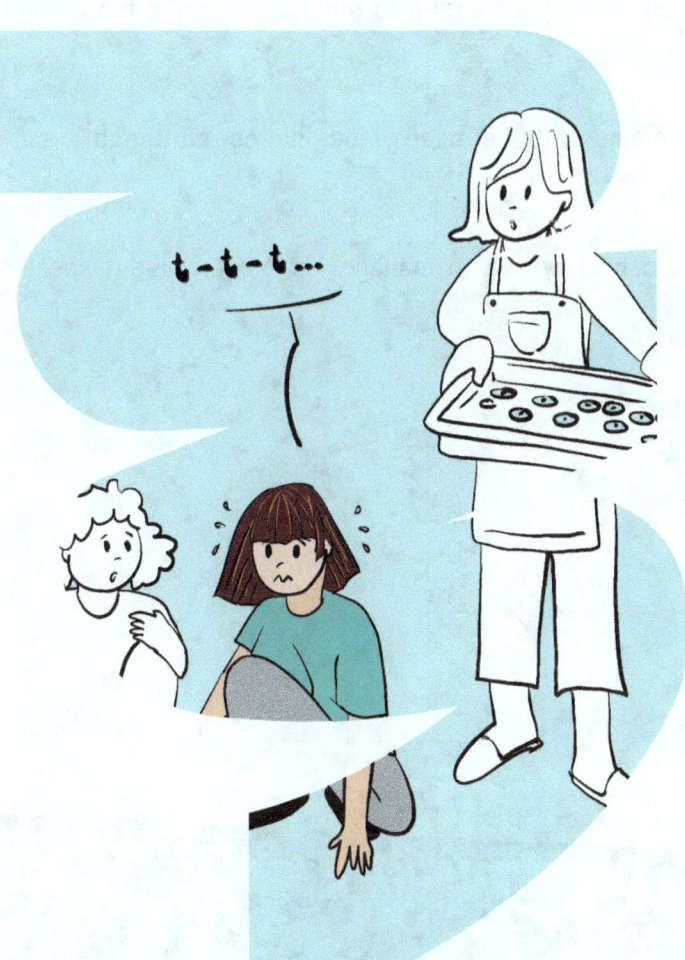

15 Story analysis

Questions...

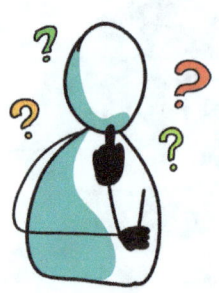

1. On a scale of 1 to 10 (1 = very little, 10 = very much), how much do you think Mary stutters?

2. What thoughts went through Mary's mind when she was trying to talk?

3. Did Mary notice any physical reactions to her body when she stuttered?

4. How did Mary's mom support her when she had trouble speaking?

5. Did Mary feel ashamed or embarrassed about her stuttering?

6. What thoughts did Mary have after her friend offered encouragement and support?

7. How could Mary use positive self-talk to cope with her stuttering in the future?

8. What activities could Mary engage in to practice speaking more comfortably and confidently?

9. How can Mary communicate her needs regarding her stuttering to her friends and family?

10. What strategies can Mary use to manage her anxiety about speaking in social situations?

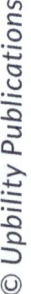

16 Unexpected meeting

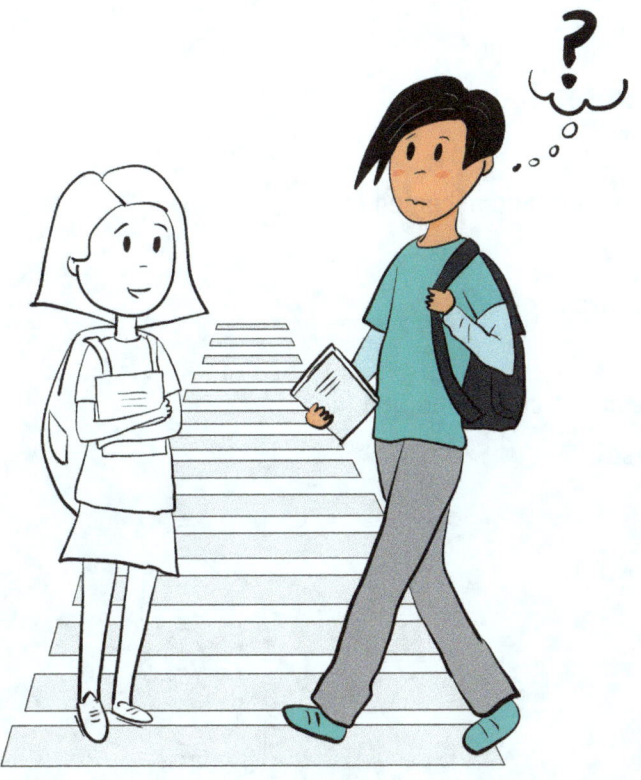

John is walking down the street when he sees Maria, a girl he knows, approaching from across. His heart is pounding at the thought of speaking to her because he stutters and always feels embarrassed about it. As Maria approaches, John wonders if he should pretend he didn't see her or start a conversation; his mind races as he struggles to find what to say. Finally, John takes a deep breath and greets Maria with a smile. "H-hi, Maria," he stammers, feeling his face flush with embarrassment.

To his surprise, Maria returns the warm smile and begins to talk to him as if nothing is wrong. John feels relieved as he realizes that his stuttering didn't bother her.

Story analysis

From John's perspective

A. Thoughts and feelings:

John may...

- Feel anxious, nervous, and ashamed of his stuttering.
- Be thinking of ways to avoid the conversation.
- Try to start the conversation and find the right words to say.

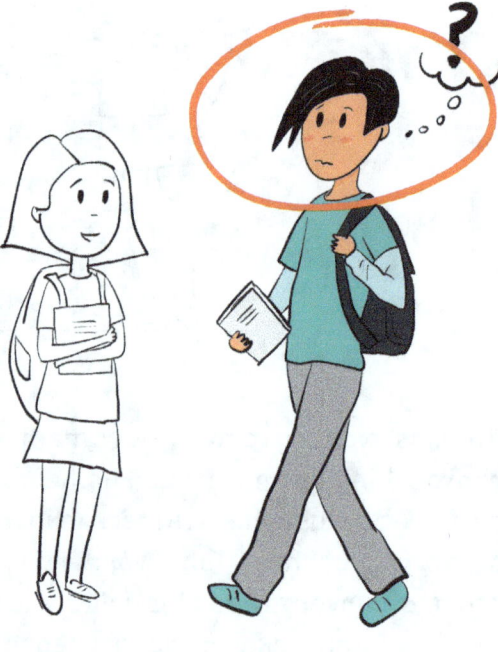

B. Possible actions:

John could...

- Pretend not to see Maria and walk away, avoiding the conversation.
- Try to start a conversation, despite his stuttering, and deal with the awkwardness.
- Take a deep breath and greet Maria with a smile to overcome his fear.

16 Story analysis

From Maria's perspective

A. Thoughts and feelings:

Maria shows understanding and compassion, as she does not react negatively to John's stuttering. She probably thinks that John's stuttering is no big deal and that she is happy talking to him.

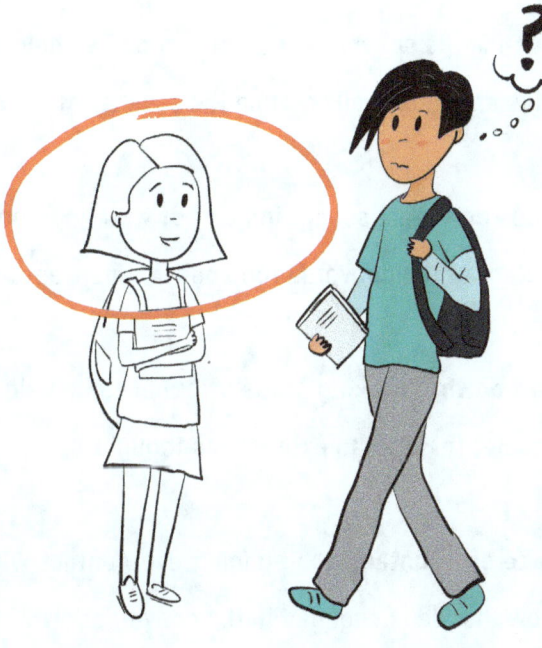

B. Possible actions:

Maria could...

- Ignore John's stuttering and continue the conversation as if nothing is happening.
- Offer encouragement or support to help John feel more comfortable.
- Perceive John's discomfort and try to change the subject to something easier for him to discuss.

Story analysis

Tips for effective communication:

John should:

Relax and breathe: Take a few deep breaths before starting a conversation to calm down and reduce stress.

Practice his speech: Regular practice can help John gain confidence in his communication skills and potentially reduce the severity of his stuttering.

Focus on the message: Instead of worrying about his stuttering, John should focus on the content of the conversation and what he wants to say.

Slow down: Speaking at a slower pace can help reduce the chances of stuttering and make it easier for John to express his thoughts.

Make eye contact: Maintaining eye contact with Maria can help build a relationship and show that he is engaged in the conversation.

Be honest about the stuttering: If John is comfortable, he can mention his stuttering beforehand, which can help him feel less self-conscious and make it easier for both parties.

© Upbility Publications

16 Story analysis

Summary

Maria's patience and active listening skills created a comfortable environment for John to express himself without the fear of criticism. Her body language and constant eye contact showed genuine interest in what John had to say, which boosted his confidence. Maria's encouraging and supportive attitude allowed John to overcome his communication anxiety gradually, and eventually, he became more comfortable starting conversations with others. Maria's behavior not only improved John's communication skills but also had a long-lasting impact on his overall self-esteem and social interactions.

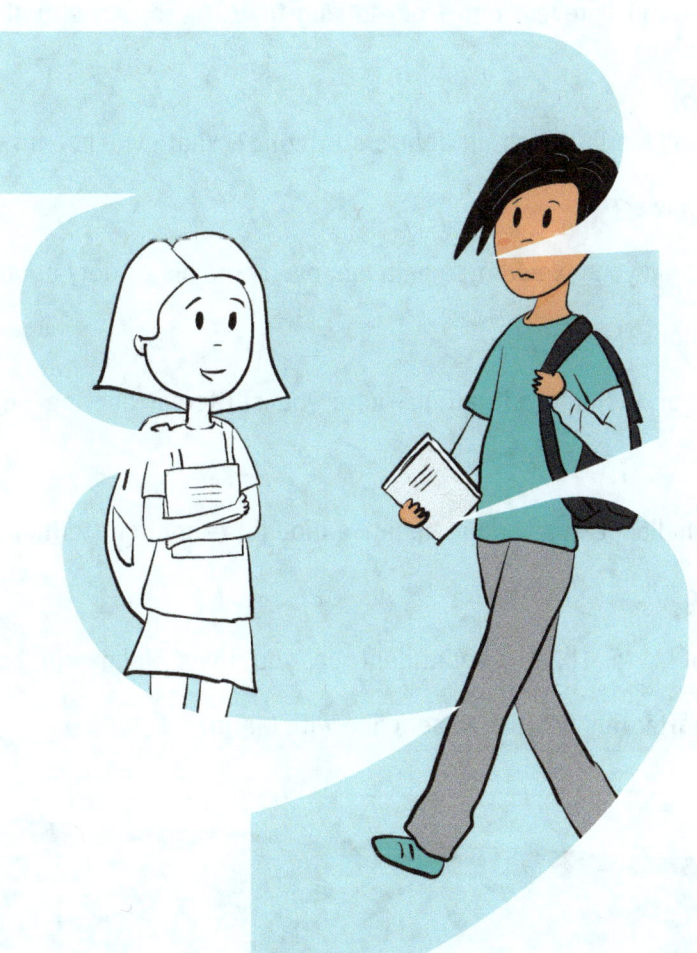

Story analysis

Questions...

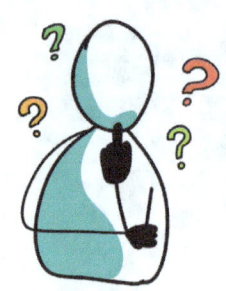

1. On a scale of 1 to 10 (1 = very little, 10 = very much), how much do you think John stutters?

2. How do you think John felt when he saw Maria approaching, and why do you think he felt that way?

3. Can you identify any negative thoughts that John may have had before he spoke to Maria? What were they?

4. How did John's feelings change after he started talking to Maria? Why do you think they changed?

5. Did John's stuttering prevent him from talking to Maria in this situation? Why or why not?

6. How do you think Maria felt about John's stuttering? What evidence do you have to support your answer?

7. What advice would you give John to help him overcome his anxiety about stuttering in social situations?

8. Can you think of a similar situation where you stuttered, but the outcome was positive?

9. How can you challenge and change negative thoughts about stuttering, as John did in this scenario?

10. On a scale of 1 to 10, how confident do you think John will be in future conversations after this positive experience with Maria?

17 The phone call

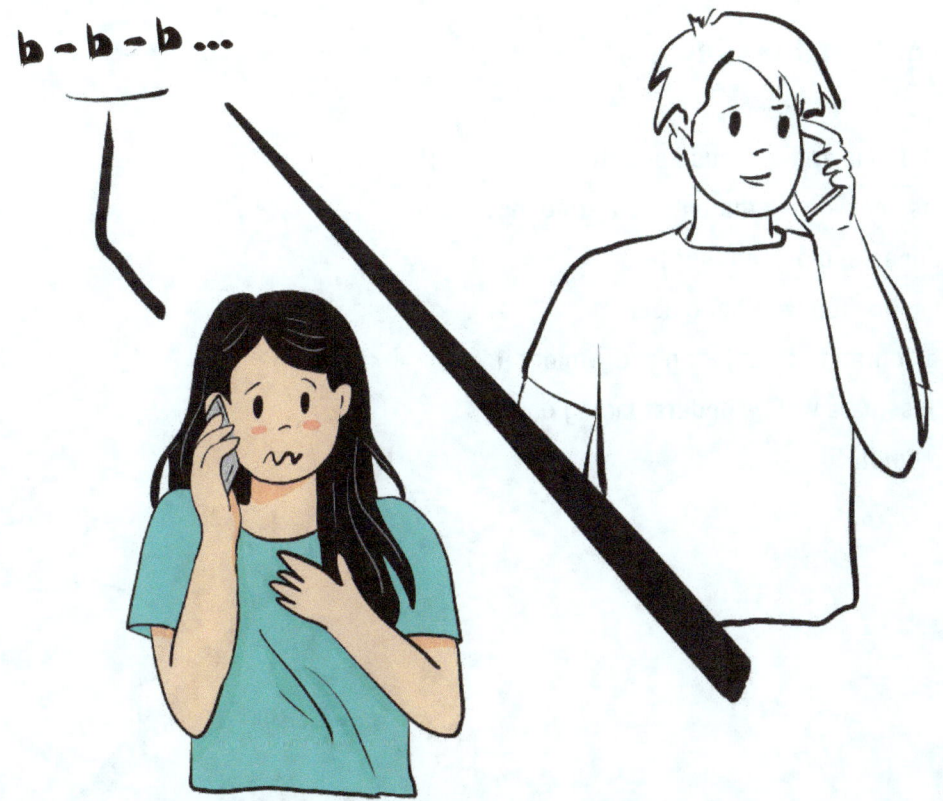

Zeta nervously dials a number on her phone, hoping her classmate won't notice her stuttering. As he picks up the phone, her heart is pounding, and her words come out with too much effort and many repetitions. However, with each passing moment, she is gaining confidence. She takes a deep breath, steadies her voice, and speaks slowly and clearly. Finally, she realizes that her stuttering isn't holding her back, and she can communicate effectively, even over the phone, albeit with a little effort and patience.

Story analysis

From Zeta's perspective

A. Thoughts and feelings:

Zeta may...

- Feel nervous and anxious about the phone call, as she worries that her stuttering may be noticed and prevent her from communicating with her classmate.

- Try to control her stuttering and wonder if her classmate will be understanding or judgmental.

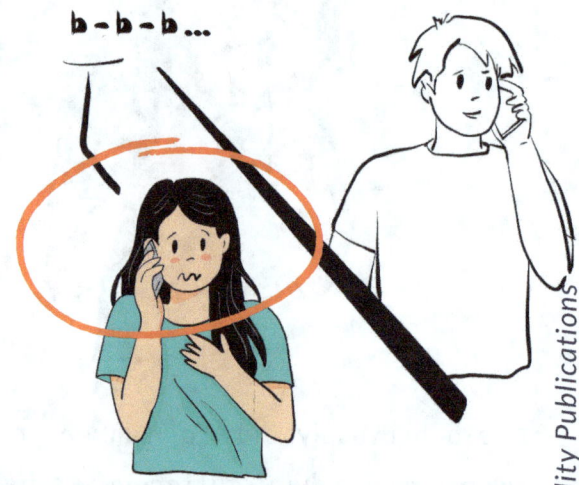

B. Possible actions:

Zeta could...

- Take deep breaths to calm herself before and during the conversation.
- Practice her speech or rehearse what she wants to say before she makes the call.
- Speak slowly and softly.
- Explain to her classmate about her stuttering and ask for patience.
- Use other methods of communication (e.g., text message or email) if she finds the phone call too difficult.

© Upbility Publications

17 Story analysis

From the classmate's perspective

A. Thoughts and feelings:

Zeta's classmate may...

- Feel confused or worried about Zeta's stuttering, initially.
- Wonder if Zeta is experiencing a temporary problem or if the stuttering occurs frequently.
- Feel relieved and impressed by Zeta's determination to communicate effectively despite her stuttering as the conversation develops and her speech improves.

B. Possible actions:

- Show empathy and patience while Zeta speaks, offering reassurance that he understands her.
- Ask if Zeta needs a minute to gather her thoughts or if there is anything he can do to help her.
- Adapt his communication to Zeta's needs, such as speaking more slowly or clearly.
- Suggest that they continue the conversation through another means if Zeta is struggling or feels uncomfortable.
- After the call, discuss the situation with Zeta to understand her experience and explore how he can support her in future communications.

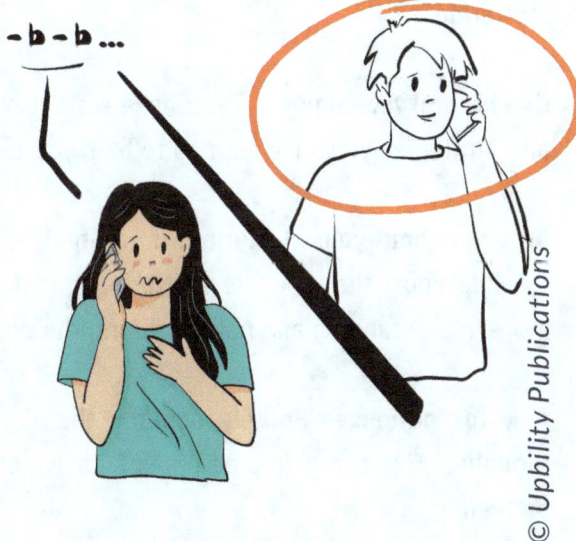

Story analysis

Tips for effective communication:

Be prepared: Before making or receiving a phone call, take some time to gather your thoughts and think about what you want to say. This can help reduce anxiety and make the conversation smoother.

Practice deep breathing: Slow breathing can help calm you and control your speech. Practice deep breathing techniques before and during the phone call to keep yourself focused.

Speak slowly and softly: Take your time while speaking and try to focus on each word individually. This can help you maintain control of your speech and reduce the chances of stuttering.

Use helpful techniques: If you have worked with a speech therapist, apply the techniques and strategies you have learned to help you control your stuttering during the phone call.

Be open about your stuttering: If you feel comfortable, let the person on the other end of the line know that you are stuttering. Most people will appreciate your honesty and be more understanding and patient during the conversation.

Ask for patience: Politely ask for the listener's patience while communicating your thoughts. This can help create a supportive environment and relieve any pressure you may be feeling.

Take breaks: If you feel overwhelmed or have difficulty communicating, pause for a moment to gather your thoughts and regain your composure.

Story analysis

Tips for effective communication:

Use alternative methods of communication: If talking on the phone becomes too difficult, consider using alternative means of communication such as text messaging, email, or voicemail.

Be patient with yourself: Remember that it's okay to stutter, and don't let it define your self-esteem. Be patient with yourself and acknowledge your progress as you work to improve your communication skills.

Practice regularly: The more you practice speaking on the phone, the more comfortable you feel and the more confident you will be. Engage regularly in telephone conversations to boost your confidence and improve your communication skills.

Story analysis

Summary

In the end, Zeta's determination and persistence allowed her to overcome her anxiety about phone conversations. Through practice, patience, and various communication strategies, she gained more confidence and effectiveness in expressing herself, even with her stuttering. Zeta's journey proved the power of patience and self-acceptance, showing that challenges can be turned into opportunities for growth. As her communication skills improved, so did her relationships with her peers, who admired and supported her. Zeta's story is an inspiring reminder that anyone can overcome obstacles and achieve personal success with the right mindset and approach.

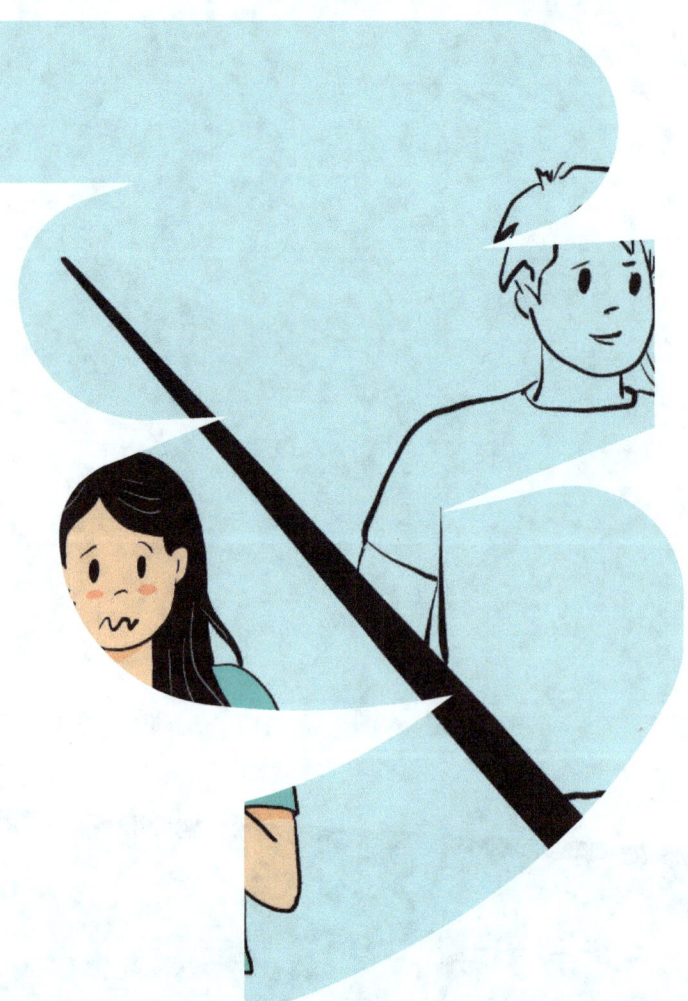

Story analysis

Questions...

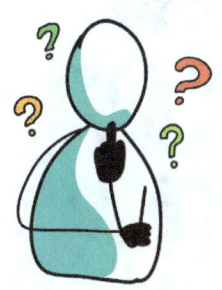

1. On a scale of 1 to 10 (1 = very little, 10 = very much), how much do you think Zeta stutters?

2. How do you think Zeta felt when she first dialed the phone number?

3. Can you identify Zeta's thoughts that could have contributed to her initial anxiety and stuttering?

4. What strategies did Zeta use to help her gain confidence while talking on the phone?

5. What was the turning point for Zeta when she realized that her stuttering was not holding her back?

6. How do you think Zeta's classmate may have reacted or felt during the phone call?

7. Can you think of a time when you faced a similar situation? How did you handle it?

8. What could you learn from Zeta's experience and apply to your communication challenges?

9. In the future, how could Zeta prepare herself for similar situations so that she feels more confident from the start?

10. How can practicing patience and self-compassion help someone who stutters when communicating with others?

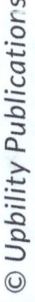

18 Playing with friends

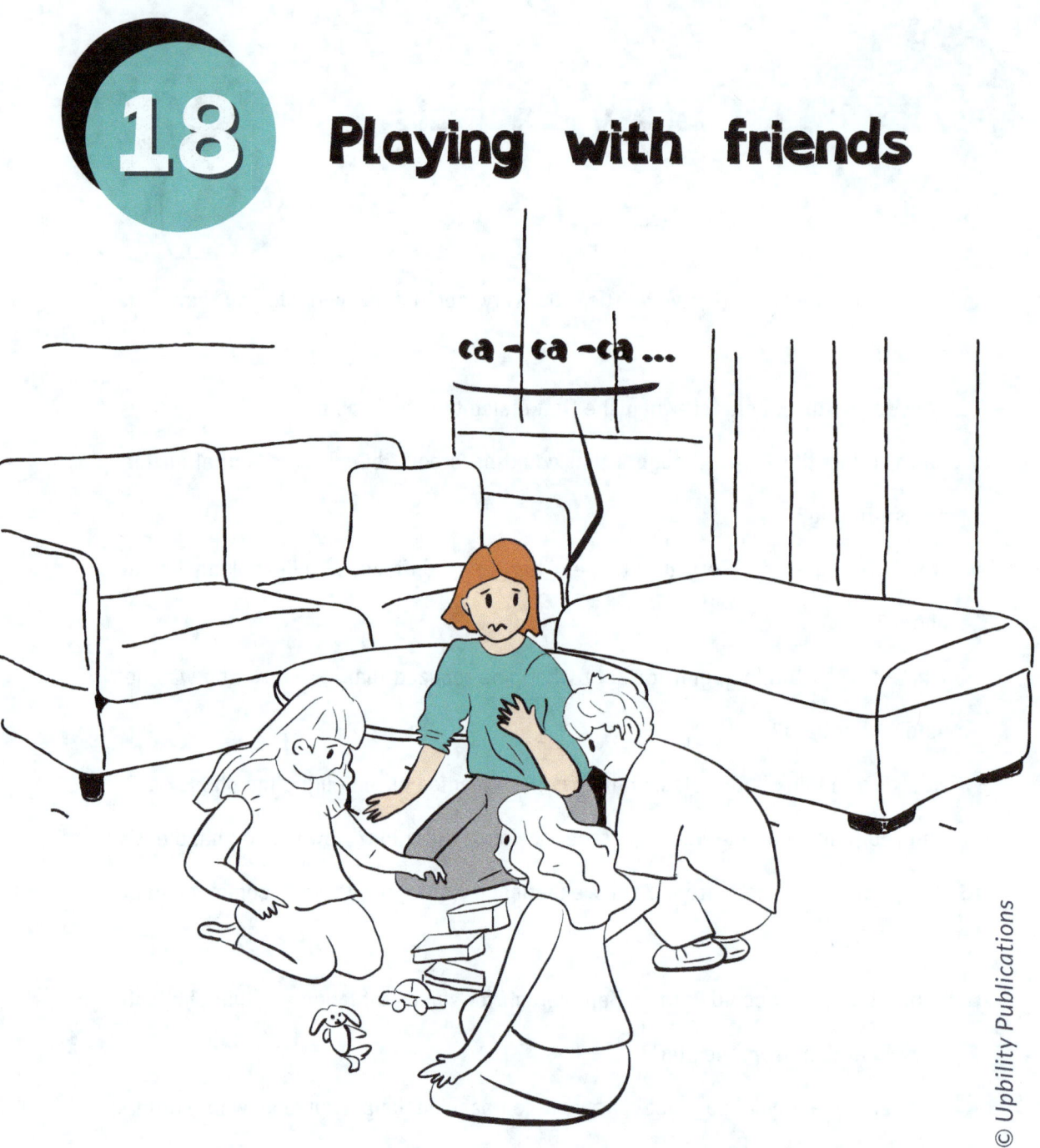

ca - ca -ca ...

Lola, a nine-year-old girl who occasionally stutters, visits a friend's house to play with other children. Lola tries to participate in the game actively, but her stuttering makes it difficult for her to speak, so she feels left out.

Story analysis

From Lola's perspective

A. Thoughts and feelings:

Lola may...

- Feel excluded and frustrated, as her stuttering keeps her from participating in the game and having a conversation with her friends.
- Think about how to better express her thoughts and be more involved in her friends' activities.

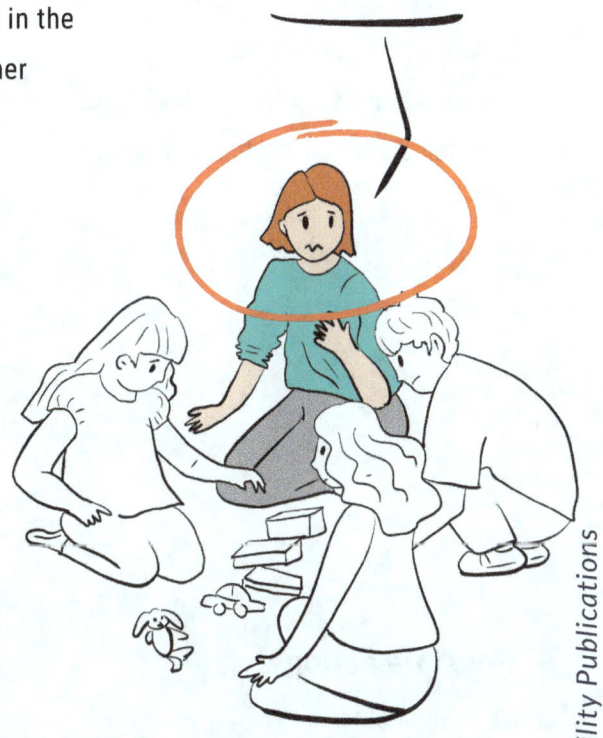

B. Possible actions:

Lola could:

- Try to speak more slowly or more softly to control her stuttering.
- Use non-verbal communication, such as gestures or facial expressions, to express herself.
- Look for alternative ways to participate, such as writing or drawing.
- Open up to her friends about her feelings and ask for their understanding and support.

Story analysis

From Lola's friend's perspective

A. Thoughts and feelings:

Lola's friend may...

- Feel concerned, show empathy, or even experience guilt for not including Lola more in their game and conversation.
- Consider ways to help Lola feel more included and comfortable in their presence.

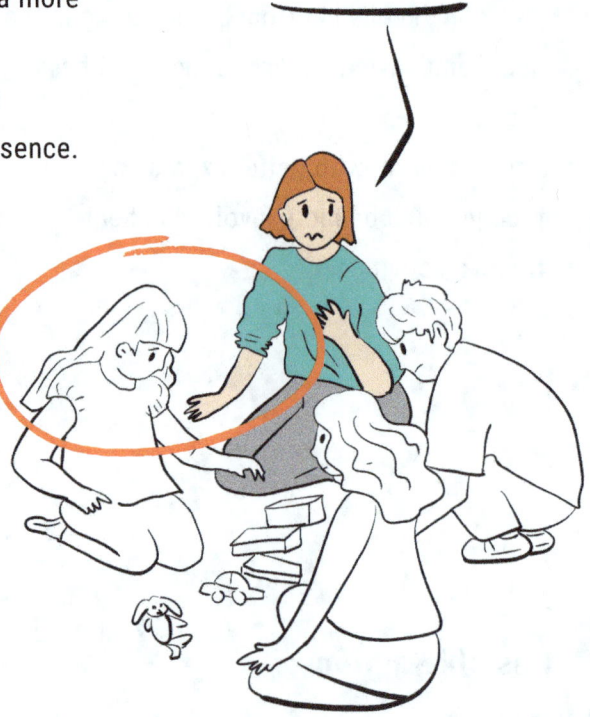

ca - ca -ca ...

B. Possible actions:

Lola's friend could:

- Include Lola in the conversation by asking her for her opinion.
- Adapt the game to be more inclusive, considering Lola's communication difficulties.
- Offer support and reassurance to Lola, helping her to feel more comfortable.
- Encourage other friends to be patient and understanding of Lola's stuttering.

Story analysis

From the perspective of bystanders

A. Thoughts and feelings:

Bystanders may...

- Feel a mixture of emotions such as curiosity, concern, or even discomfort as they observe the situation.

- Think about how they would handle a similar situation or how they can help Lola feel more included.

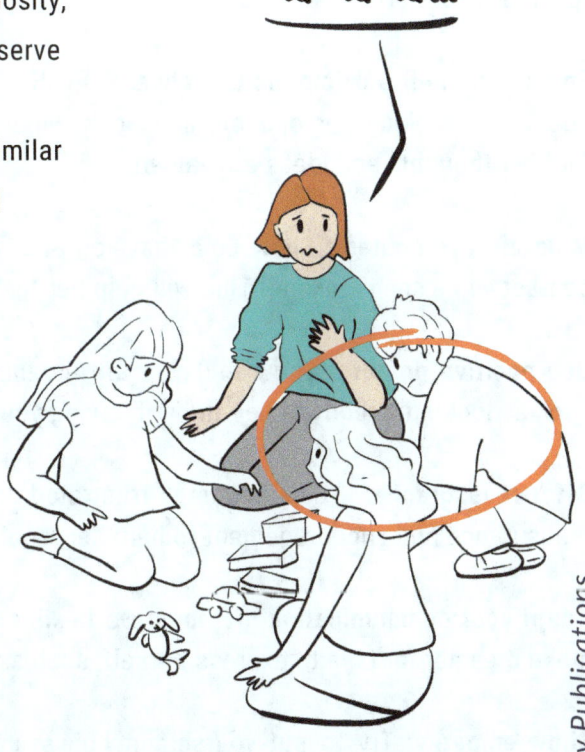

ca – ca –ca ...

B. Possible actions:

Bystanders could...

- Start the conversation and try to include Lola, making her feel more welcome.

- Make suggestions about how to adapt the game or conversation to get Lola more involved.

- Share their experiences with stuttering or communication challenges to help Lola feel less alone.

- Encourage an open discussion about stuttering, promoting empathy and understanding between group members.

18 Story analysis

Tips for effective communication:

Be patient and understanding: When talking to Lola, give her time to express her thoughts without interrupting or completing her sentences. Patience and understanding will help her feel more comfortable and supported.

Encourage her participation: Actively involve Lola in the discussion by asking her questions, seeking her opinion, and acknowledging her contribution. This will show her that her thoughts and ideas are valued.

Maintain eye contact: Show Lola that you are engaged and listening by maintaining eye contact while she is talking. This will help her feel more comfortable and confident.

Use positive posture: Show that you are listening and caring by using positive posture, such as looking directly at her and not having your arms crossed.

Offer reassurance: If Lola becomes frustrated or embarrassed about her stuttering, offer reassurance and encouragement to help her regain her confidence.

Adapt your communication methods: Be flexible and consider alternative ways that might make it easier for Lola to express herself, such as writing, drawing, or using gestures.

Show empathy: Try to put yourself in Lola's shoes and understand the challenges she faces due to her stuttering. This way, you will become a more compassionate and effective listener.

Create a welcoming environment: Encourage an atmosphere where everyone's input is valued and respected, ensuring that Lola and others with communication difficulties feel included and supported.

Story analysis

Tips for effective communication:

Educate yourself and others: Learn more about stuttering and its effects on communication. Share this information with others to promote understanding and reduce misconceptions or stereotypes.

Offer support: Let Lola know you are there for her and willing to help her overcome communication challenges. You can help her gain confidence and strengthen her communication skills by offering your support and understanding.

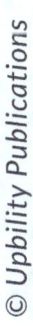

18 Story analysis

Summary

In conclusion, Lola's story highlights the importance of understanding, patience, and empathy when interacting with people facing communication difficulties such as stuttering. As her friends and bystanders become more aware of her condition, they learn to adjust their communication and create a more inclusive and supportive environment for Lola. Over time, with the encouragement and understanding of her friends, Lola gains confidence and finds new ways to express herself and participate in conversations and games. As a result, she no longer feels excluded, and her friendships become more meaningful.

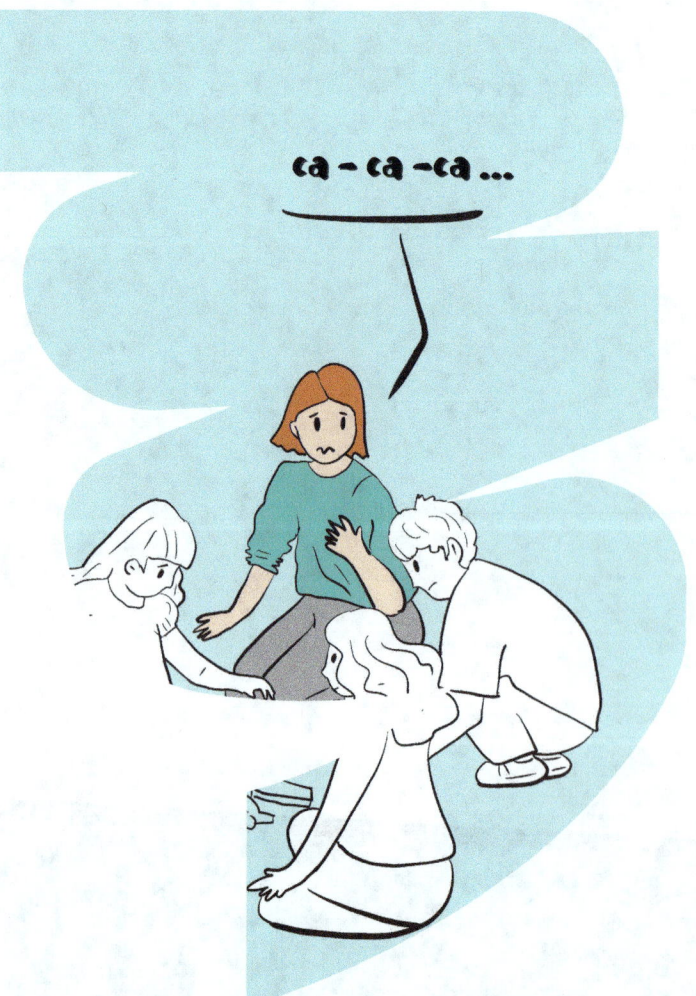

18 Story analysis

Questions...

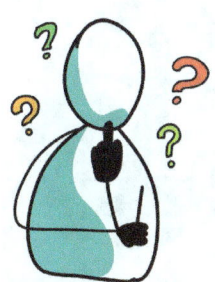

1. On a scale of 1 to 10 (1=slightly, 10=very much), how much do you think Lola stutters?

2. How does Lola feel when she stutters during the conversation?

3. What thoughts go through Lola's mind when she cannot fully participate in the conversation?

4. How do Lola's friends react to her stuttering?

5. Can Lola identify specific situations or triggers that make her stuttering more intense?

6. How would Lola like her friends to react or support her when she stutters?

7. What are some coping strategies or techniques that Lola has tried to manage her stuttering?

8. Are there any activities or situations in which Lola feels more confident in her speech?

9. How does Lola's stuttering affect her overall self-esteem and self-image?

10. What are some small steps Lola can take to improve her communication and feel more included in conversations with her friends?

19 I wish I were different

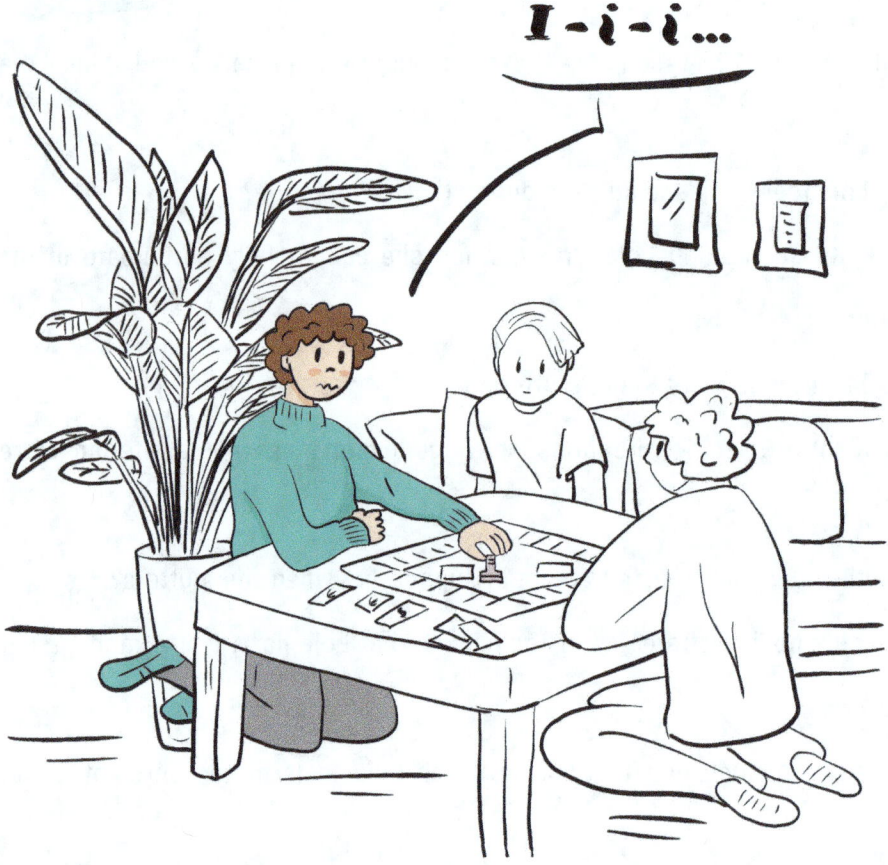

Pete places his pawn on the Monopoly board, his heart pounding as he realizes he's the winner. He feels his friends staring at him as they wait for him to speak. But when he tries to say something, the words are stuck in his throat, and he stutters. His friends look away awkwardly, not knowing how to react. Pete feels the familiar frustration as he realizes he cannot enjoy his victory. He wishes he were like everyone else, effortlessly speaking his mind without second thoughts.

19 Story analysis

From Pete's perspective

A. Thoughts and feelings:

Pete may feel...

- Excited and proud to have won the game. However, when he tries to speak, he experiences anxiety and frustration because he stutters and cannot express his feelings as he would like to.
- Jealous of those who can speak effortlessly and wish he could be more like them.

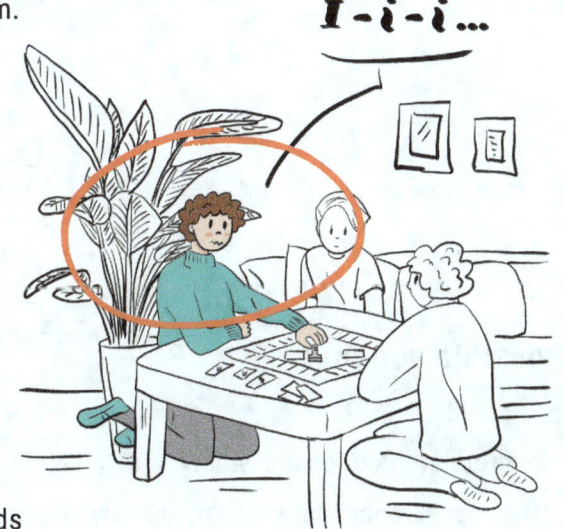

B. Possible actions:

Pete could:

- Speak again, trying to overcome his stuttering.
- Remain silent, hoping that his friends will understand his feelings.
- Use non-verbal signs to express his excitement and happiness.
- Change the subject to reduce tension.
- Seek help or therapy to improve his communication skills in the future.

19 Story analysis

From the friends' perspective

A. Thoughts and feelings:

Pete's friends may...

- Feel disappointed for their defeat in the game and empathy for Pete's struggle with stuttering at the same time.

- Not be sure how to react or support Pete in this situation.

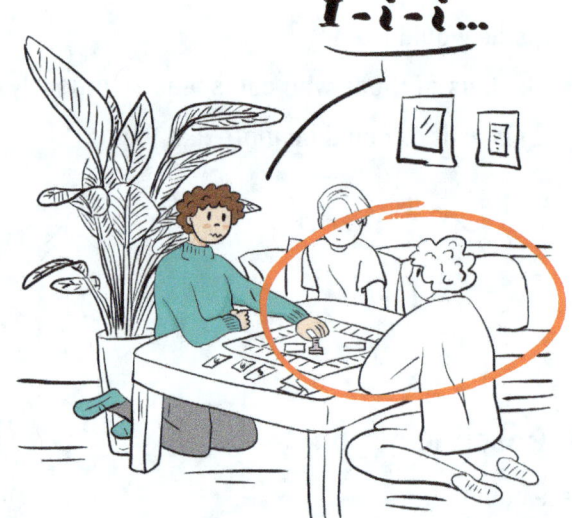

B. Possible actions:

Friends could:

- Congratulate Pete on his victory, making him feel recognized and appreciated.

- Offer reassurance and support, acknowledging Pete's difficulty in speaking.

- Guide the conversation to a more comfortable topic.

- Encourage Pete to express himself in other ways, such as writing or gestures.

- Discuss the situation with Pete afterward to offer support and understanding.

19 Story analysis

From the perspective of bystanders

A. Thoughts and feelings:

- Bystanders may feel sympathetic for Pete's struggle and awkward due to the unexpected turn of events.
- They may also be unsure how to react or whether to intervene.

B. Possible actions:

Bystanders could:

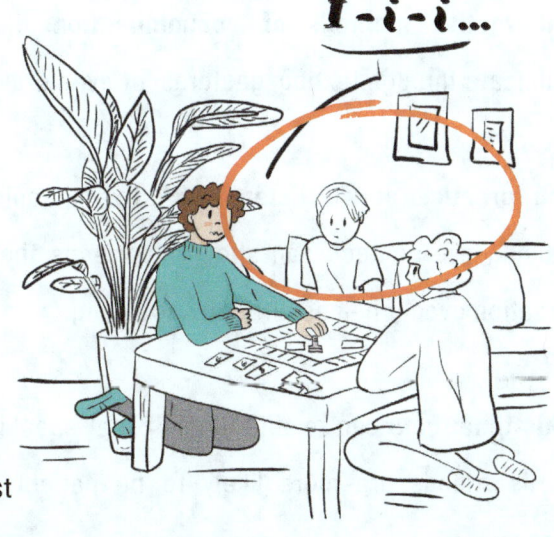

- Offer support and encouragement to Pete.
- Remain silent and let things unfold, giving Pete and his friends space to manage the situation.
- Redirect the conversation, or suggest a new activity to ease the tension.
- Share their experience with communication challenges, helping Pete to feel less isolated and more understood.
- Offer suggestions for speech therapy or support groups if they feel it's appropriate and have such information.

Story analysis

Tips for effective communication:

Pete should:

Be open and honest: He can share his feelings and struggles with stuttering, helping his friends to better understand his situation. This can reinforce empathy and create a supportive environment.

Use alternative methods of communication: If speech is a challenge, Pete can communicate through texting, gestures, or even drawings to express himself.

He can practice active listening: Active listening practices, such as nodding and maintaining eye contact, can show his friends that he is present and interested in the conversation even if he has difficulty speaking.

Take his time: Pete can remind himself that speaking slowly and pausing if necessary is okay. His friends are more likely to be patient and understanding if they know his challenges.

Develop coping strategies: Pete can practice relaxation techniques, breathing exercises, or other strategies to manage his anxiety and stuttering during conversations.

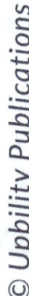

Story analysis

Tips for effective communication:

Seek professional help: Pete may consider seeking help from a speech and language therapist or joining a support group to improve his communication skills and gain confidence.

Focus on non-verbal cues: Pete can improve his non-verbal communication skills, such as facial expressions, body language, and eye contact, to improve his overall communication with his friends.

Encourage open dialogue: Pete can create a safe space for his friends to discuss their challenges and concerns, fostering an environment of understanding and support.

Be patient with himself: Pete should remember that effective communication is an ongoing process, and being patient and kind to himself as he works through his difficulties is important.

Surround himself with supportive friends: Creating a circle of friends who understand and support him can help him feel more comfortable and confident in his communication.

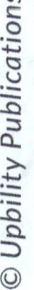

Story analysis

Summary

Despite his win, Pete finds it difficult to fully enjoy and share his excitement with others due to his speech difficulty. However, by being honest with his friends, exploring alternative methods of communication, and seeking support, Pete can work towards improving his communication skills and building stronger bonds. By feeling more confident in himself, he can accomplish a lot. As Pete navigates these experiences, he needs to remain patient and gentle with himself, recognizing that growth and progress take time and effort.

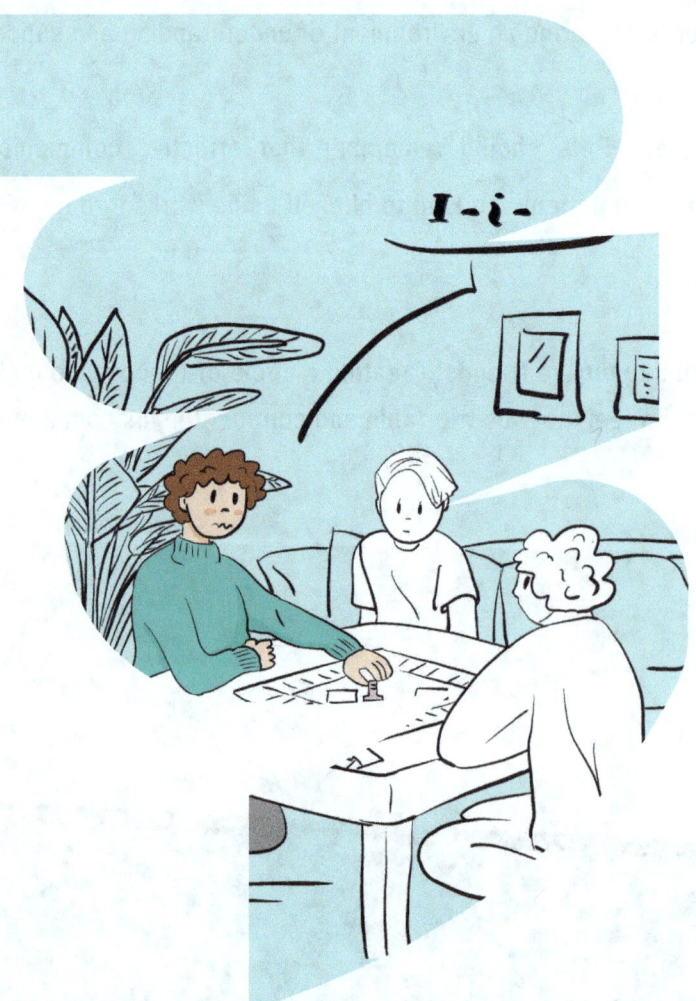

19 Story analysis

Questions...

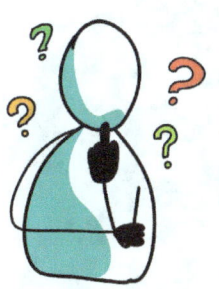

1. On a scale of 1 to 10 (1=slightly, 10=very much), how much do you think Pete stutters?

2. On a scale of 1 to 10, where would you rank your stuttering?

3. Do you think Pete's friends judge him because of his stuttering? Why or why not?

4. How do you think Pete feels when he can't express his excitement? Can you identify with his feelings?

5. What positive qualities does Pete have that his friends might appreciate despite his stuttering?

6. How might Pete's friends support him when he has difficulty speaking during a conversation?

7. What coping strategies could Pete use to manage his stuttering and anxiety in similar situations?

8. If you were in Pete's shoes, what would you want your friends to do or say to make you feel more comfortable?

9. How could Pete change his thoughts and beliefs about his stuttering to reduce the impact on his daily life and social interactions?

10. Can you think of any role models or famous people who stutter and who have succeeded? How might their experiences inspire Pete and others who stutter?

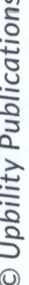

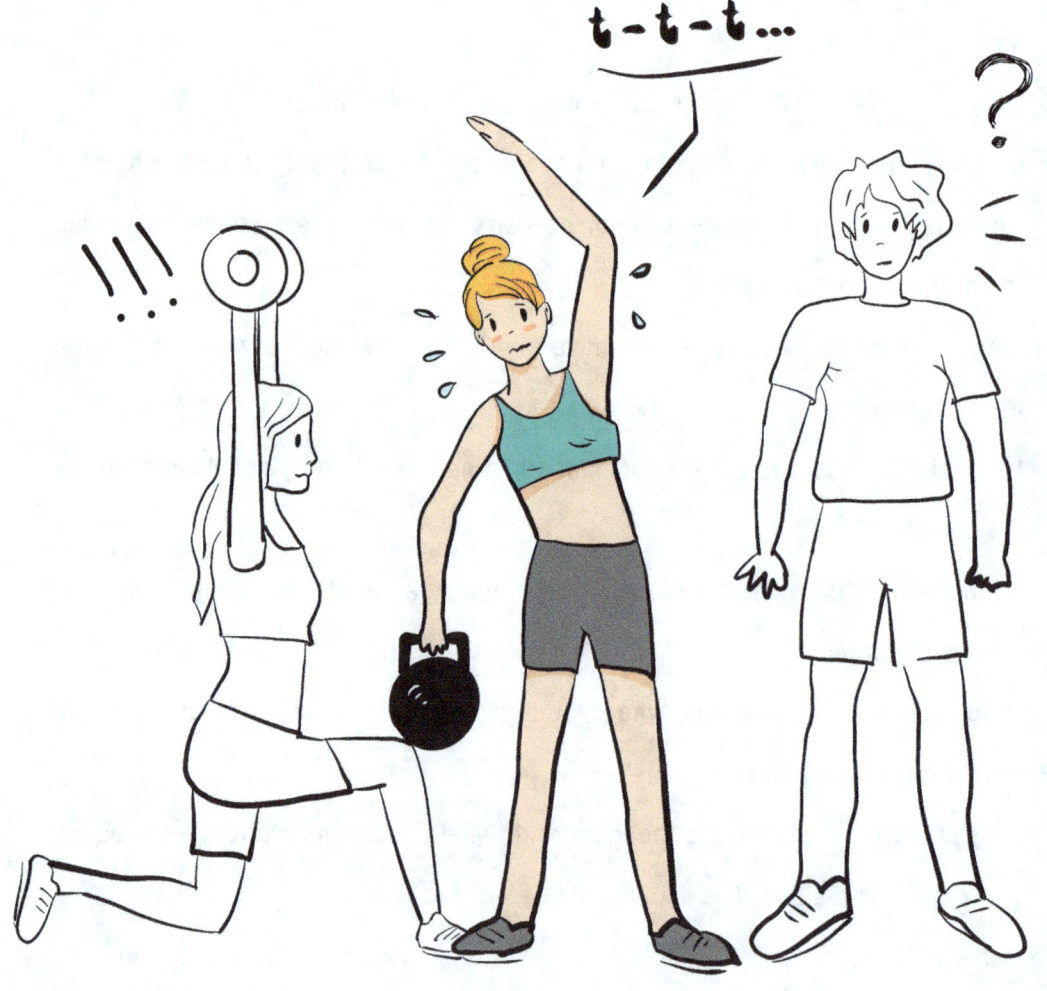

Nicole goes to the gym every afternoon. Today she started a new exercise program and wants to ask her trainer if she is executing her drills correctly. But as soon as she opens her mouth to speak, she stutters and feels her face flush with embarrassment.

Story analysis

From Nicole's perspective

A. Thoughts and feelings:

Nicole may feel...

- Embarrassed and frustrated because she stuttered when she tried to ask her trainer for help with her new exercise program.
- Anxious about speaking up again in the future.

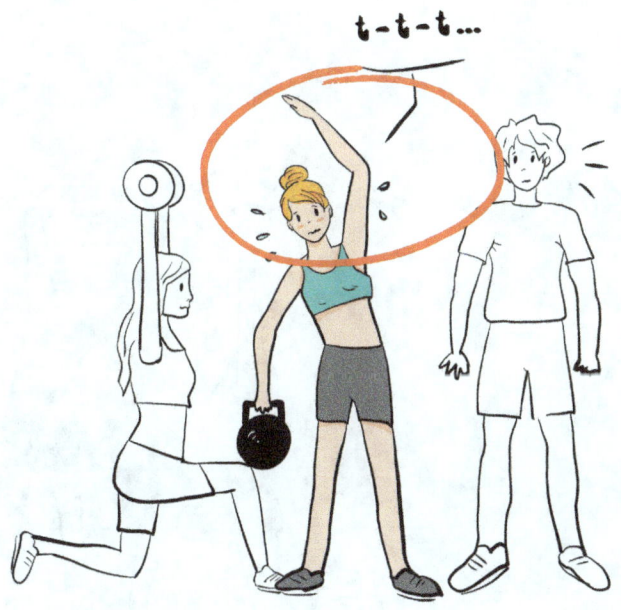

B. Possible actions:

- Nicole could be reluctant to ask for help again or avoid going to the gym because of her embarrassment.
- She could try to practice her speech or seek speech therapy to address her stuttering.

Story analysis

From the trainer's perspective

A. Thoughts and feelings:

The trainer may...

- Observe Nicole's stuttering and sympathize with her condition.
- Feel responsible for helping Nicole with her new exercise program.

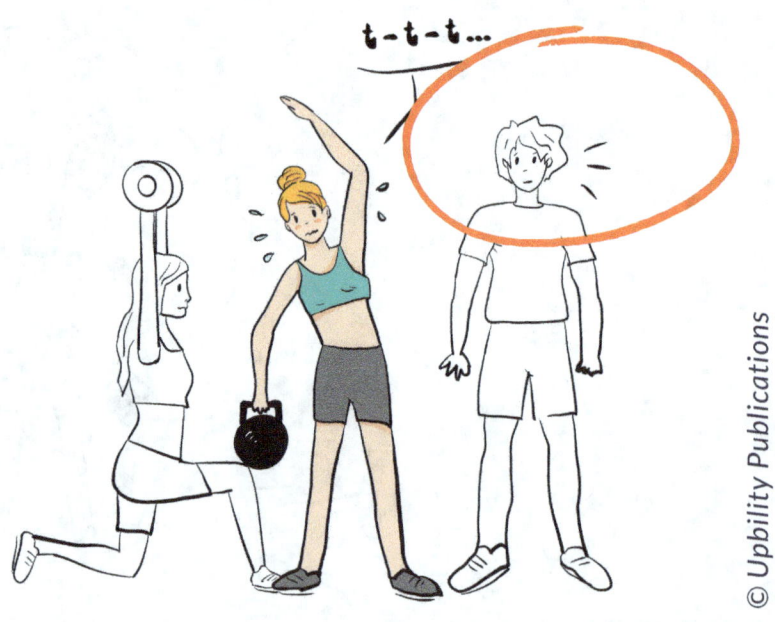

B. Possible actions:

The trainer could offer guidance and feedback on the new exercise program or take extra time to listen to her to help her feel more comfortable with her speech.

Story analysis

From the perspective of bystanders

A. Thoughts and feelings:

Bystanders may feel...

- Various emotions, such as empathy, curiosity, or indifference to Nicole's stuttering.
- Sorry for her, while others may not notice her stuttering or care.

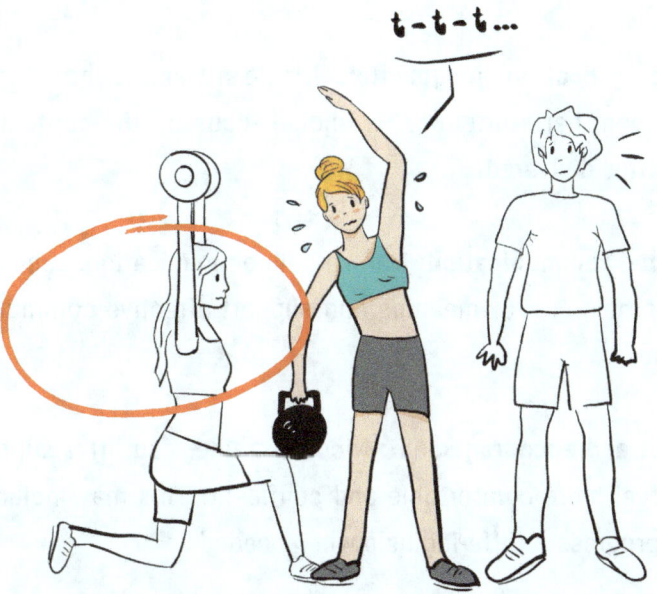

t-t-t...

B. Possible actions:

- Bystanders can offer encouragement and support to Nicole.
- They can continue their training without paying attention to the situation.
- Some may be curious about the stuttering and seek information or resources to better understand it.

Story analysis

Tips for effective communication:

Patience and understanding: It is important for Nicole's trainer to be patient and understanding when communicating with her. He should give her time to express herself and avoid interrupting or finishing her sentences.

Actively listen: Nicole and her trainer should actively listen to each other to ensure clear communication. This means paying attention to what the other person is saying and asking for clarification if necessary.

Avoid being critical or judgmental: Nicole's trainer should avoid being critical or judgmental about her stuttering. He should focus on the content of her message rather than the way it is delivered.

Use non-verbal communication: Non-verbal communication, such as facial expressions or gestures, can help convey meaning and support effective communication between Nicole and her trainer.

Offer support and encouragement: Nicole's trainer can offer support and encouragement to help her feel more comfortable and confident. This may include positive feedback on her training progress or offering help when needed.

Be flexible: Nicole's trainer must be flexible and adaptable when communicating with her. He may need to adjust his approach based on Nicole's needs and preferences.

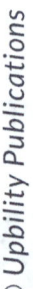

20 Story analysis

Summary

Effective communication between Nicole and her trainer can be important, who can offer support and encouragement to help her feel more comfortable and confident. With patience, understanding, and flexibility, her trainer and Nicole can work together to create a safe and supportive environment where she can achieve her fitness goals and maintain good communication skills.

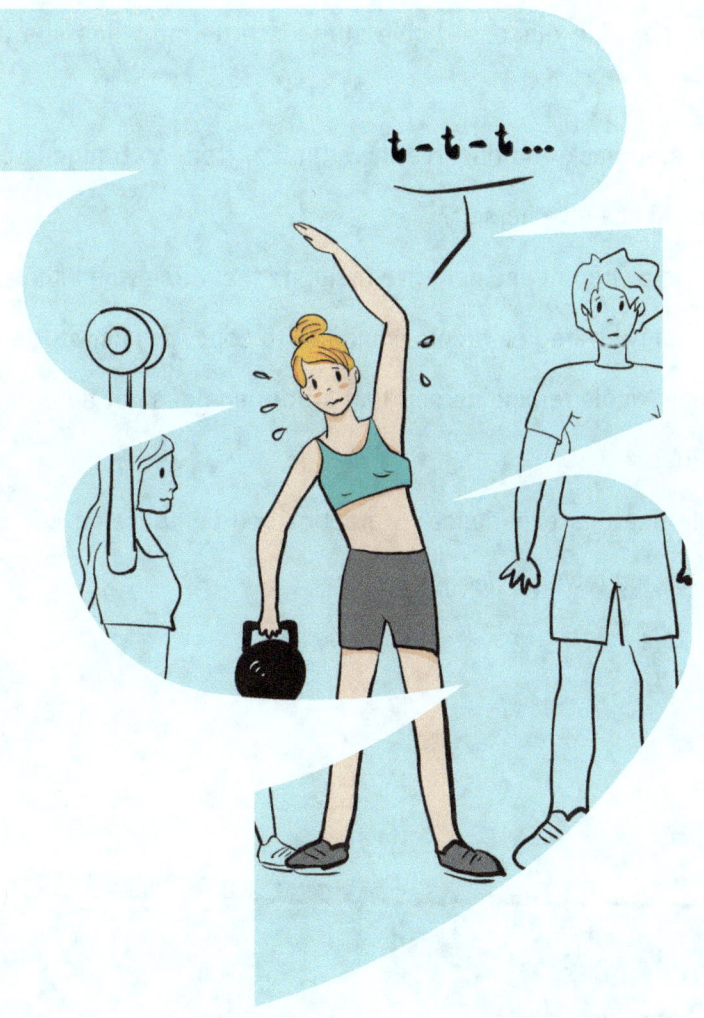

Story analysis

Questions...

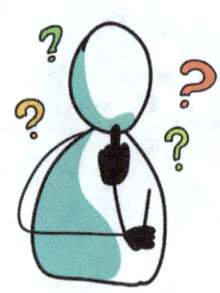

1. On a scale of 1 to 10 (1 = very little, 10 = very much), how much do you think Nicole stutters?

2. How does Nicole feel when she starts to stutter? Can you describe the emotions she might be experiencing?

3. What thoughts might go through Nicole's mind when she begins to stutter in front of her trainer?

4. How do you think Nicole's trainer might react to her stuttering? What makes you believe that?

5. What are some possible reasons Nicole started stuttering when she tried to ask her question?

6. If Nicole could step back and observe the situation from a stranger's perspective, what advice would she give herself?

7. How could Nicole overcome the negative thoughts that arise when she stutters?

8. Can you think of any strategies Nicole could use to cope with her stuttering?

9. In what ways can Nicole remind herself that stuttering does not determine her self-esteem or abilities?

10. How can Nicole use this experience to practice self-compassion and acceptance and continue working towards her gym goals?

© Upbility Publications

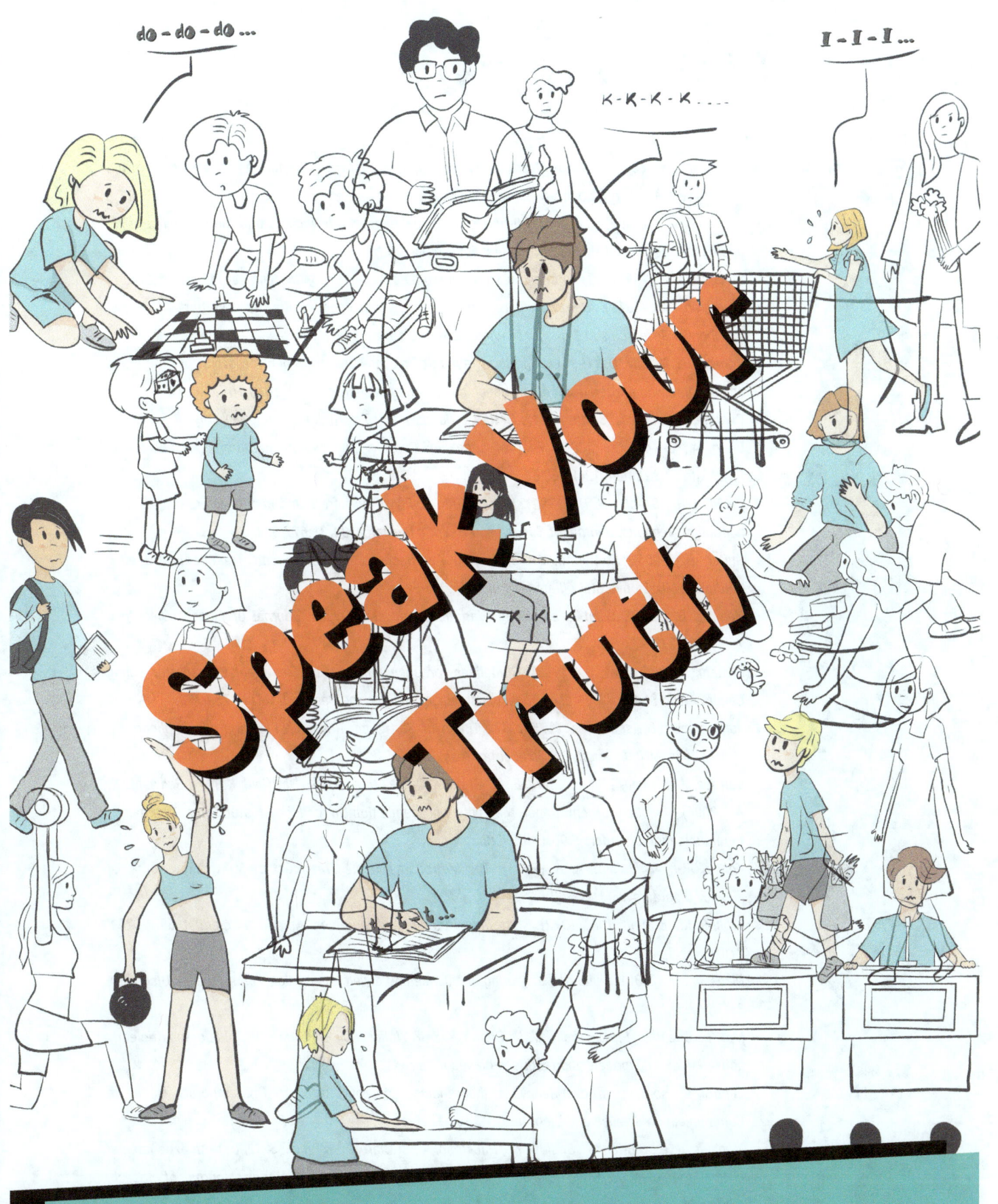

Bibliography

- *American Speech-Language-Hearing Association. (n.d.). Stuttering. Retrieved from https://www.asha.org/public/speech/disorders/stuttering/*
- *Andrews, G., & Guitar, B. (1975). Stuttering: A review of research findings and theories circa 1975. Journal of Speech and Hearing Disorders, 40(3), 408-426.*
- *Bloodstein, O. (1995). A Handbook on Stuttering (5th ed.). San Diego, CA: Singular Publishing Group.*
- *Blomgren, M. (2013). Behavioral treatments for children and adults who stutter: A review. Psychology Research and Behavior Management, 6, 9-19.*
- *Boberg, E., & Kully, D. (1994). Long-term results of an intensive treatment program for adults and adolescents who stutter. Journal of Speech and Hearing Research, 37(5), 1050-1059.*
- *Conture, E. G. (2001). Stuttering: Its Nature, Diagnosis, and Treatment. Boston, MA: Allyn & Bacon.*
- *Craig, A., & Tran, Y. (2006). Fear of speaking: Chronic anxiety and stammering. Advances in Psychiatric Treatment, 12(1), 63-68.*
- *De Nil, L. F., & Abbs, J. H. (1991). Kinaesthetic acuity of stutterers and nonstutterers for oral and nonoral movements. Journal of Speech and Hearing Research, 34(3), 677-684.*
- *Guitar, B. (2006). Stuttering: An Integrated Approach to Its Nature and Treatment (3rd ed.). Baltimore, MD: Lippincott Williams & Wilkins.*
- *Ham, R. E. (1990). What is stuttering: Variations and stereotypes. Journal of Fluency Disorders, 15(4), 259-273.*
- *Ingham, R. J., & Riley, G. (1998). Guidelines for Documentation of Treatment Efficacy for Young Children Who Stutter. Journal of Speech, Language, and Hearing Research, 41(4), 753-770.*
- *Johnson, W., & Associates. (1959). The Onset of Stuttering: Research Findings and Implications. Minneapolis, MN: University of Minnesota Press.*
- *Karrass, J., Walden, T. A., Conture, E. G., Graham, C. G., Arnold, H. S., Hartfield, K. N., & Schwenk, K. A. (2006). Relation of emotional reactivity and regulation to childhood stuttering. Journal of Communication Disorders, 39(6), 402-423.*
- *Kehoe, T. D., & Mallard, A. R. (2001). The Metronome in the Treatment of Stuttering. Journal of Fluency Disorders, 26(1), 45-60.*
- *Kroll, R. M., & Klein, J. F. (1972). Stuttering: Theories and therapies. American Scientist, 60(2), 209-215.*
- *Månsson, H. (2000). Childhood stuttering: Incidence and development. Journal of Fluency Disorders, 25(1), 47-57.*
- *Max, L., Guenther, F. H., Gracco, V. L., Ghosh, S. S., & Wallace, M. E. (2004). Unstable or insufficiently activated internal models and feedback-biased motor*
- *control as sources of dysfluency: A theoretical model of stuttering. Contemporary Issues in Communication Science and Disorders, 31, 105-122.*
- *Menzies, R. G., O'Brian, S., Onslow, M., Packman, A., St Clare, T., & Block, S. (2008). An experimental clinical trial of a cognitive-behavior therapy package for chronic stuttering. Journal of Speech, Language, and Hearing Research, 51(6), 1451-1464.*

- Miller, S., & Watson, B. C. (1992). The relationship between communication attitude, anxiety, and depression in stutterers and nonstutterers. *Journal of Speech and Hearing Research, 35(4)*, 789-798.
- Nippold, M. A. (2012). Stuttering and language ability in children: Questioning the connection. *American Journal of Speech-Language Pathology, 21(3)*, 183-196.
- O'Donnell, J. J., & Prutting, C. A. (1991). Integrating social and nonsocial approaches to the treatment of stuttering. *Journal of Fluency Disorders, 16(1)*, 1-17.
- Onslow, M., & O'Brian, S. (2011). The Lidcombe Program of early stuttering intervention. *Seminars in Speech and Language, 32(4)*, 263-273.
- Packman, A., & Kuhn, L. (2009). Looking for the cause of stuttering: Are we any closer? *Folia Phoniatrica et Logopaedica, 61(5)*, 245-253.
- Perkins, W. H. (1990). What is stuttering? *Journal of Speech and Hearing Disorders, 55(3)*, 370-382.
- Ratner, N. B. (2005). Evidence-based practice in stuttering: Some questions to consider. *Journal of Fluency Disorders, 30(3)*, 163-188.
- Riley, G. D. (1994). *Stuttering Severity Instrument for Children and Adults (SSI-3) (3rd ed.).* Austin, TX: Pro-Ed.
- Silverman, F. H. (1996). *Stuttering and other fluency disorders (3rd ed.).* Boston, MA: Allyn & Bacon.
- Smith, A. (1999). Stuttering: A unified approach to a multifactorial, dynamic disorder. In N. B. Ratner & E. C. Healey (Eds.), *Stuttering Research and Practice: Bridging the Gap* (pp. 27-44). Mahwah, NJ: Lawrence Erlbaum Associates.
- Smith, A., & Kelly, E. (1997). Stuttering: A dynamic, multifactorial model. In R. F. Curlee & G. M. Siegel (Eds.), *Nature and Treatment of Stuttering: New Directions* (2nd ed., pp. 204-217). Boston, MA: Allyn & Bacon.
- Starkweather, C. W., & Givens-Ackerman, J. (1997). *Stuttering.* Austin, TX: Pro-Ed.
- St. Louis, K. O., & Durrenberger, C. H. (1993). What communication disorders do experienced clinicians prefer not to treat? *Language, Speech, and Hearing Services in Schools, 24(2)*, 68-74.
- Van Riper, C. (1973). *The Treatment of Stuttering*
- (2nd ed.). Englewood Cliffs, NJ: Prentice-Hall.
- Van Riper, C. (1982). *The Nature of Stuttering (2nd ed.).* Englewood Cliffs, NJ: Prentice-Hall.
- Ward, D. (2013). *Stuttering and Cluttering: Frameworks for Understanding and Treatment (2nd ed.).* Hove, UK: Psychology Press.
- Webster, R. L. (1991). The role of the cerebral hemispheres in the development of stuttering. *Journal of Fluency Disorders, 16(4)*, 207-221.
- Wingate, M. E. (1964). A Standard Definition of Stuttering. *Journal of Speech and Hearing Disorders, 29(4)*, 484-489.
- Yairi, E., & Ambrose, N. G. (2005). *Early Childhood Stuttering.* Austin, TX: Pro-Ed.
- Yaruss, J. S., & Quesal, R. W. (2004). Stuttering and the International Classification of Functioning, Disability, and Health (ICF): An update. *Journal of Communication Disorders, 37(1)*, 35-52.

- Zimmermann, G. N. (1980). Stuttering: A Disorder of Movement. *Journal of Speech and Hearing Research, 23(1)*, 122-136.
- Zimmermann, G. N., & Bernstein Ratner, N. (2016). Stuttering and Related Disorders of Fluency (4th ed.). New York, NY: Thieme.
- Blood, G. W., & Blood, I. M. (2004). Bullying in adolescents who stutter: Communicative competence and self-esteem. *Contemporary Issues in Communication Science and Disorders, 31*, 69-79.
- Brundage, S. B., & Bernstein Ratner, N. (2018). Stuttering Intervention: A Collaborative Journey to Fluency Freedom (3rd ed.). Austin, TX: Pro-Ed.
- Finn, P., & Martin, R. R. (1997). Language processing and motor production in stuttering: A review of the literature. *Journal of Fluency Disorders, 22(3)*, 169-192.
- Howell, P. (2011). Recovery from Stuttering. Hove, UK: Psychology Press.
- Neumann, K., Preibisch, C., Euler, H. A., Gudenberg, A. W., & Lanfermann, H. (2003). Cortical plasticity in the treatment of stuttering. *Journal of Speech, Language, and Hearing Research, 46(1)*, 201-209.
- Runyan, C. M., & Runyan, S. E. (1986). Stuttering: A comparison of cerebral dominance for language and emotion. *Journal of Fluency Disorders, 11(4)*, 277-286.
- Sheehan, J. G. (1970). Stuttering: Research and therapy. New York, NY: Harper & Row.
- Starkweather, C. W. (2002). The epigenesis of stuttering. *Journal of Fluency Disorders, 27(4)*, 269-288.

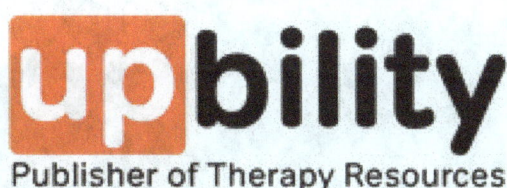

Publisher of Therapy Resources

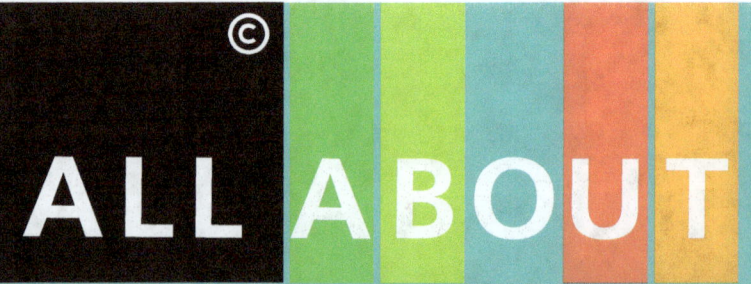

"Stuttering" is the first part of the "ALL ABOUT" series. It's an essential guide for parents, educators, therapists, and caregivers of stuttering children and adolescents.

The book offers an in-depth understanding of stuttering, a communication disorder affecting millions worldwide. It sheds light on the causes, symptoms, and types of stuttering, along with diagnostic approaches, treatment options, and practical strategies for managing this misunderstood condition. Also, it highlights the social impact of stuttering and the importance of support and education. "ALL ABOUT - Stuttering" includes 20 engaging short stories that present real-life social situations with children and adolescents who stutter, providing valuable perspectives to everyone involved.

Let's empower ourselves with the knowledge to support children and adolescents who stutter and advocate for helping them navigate the complexities of this disorder.

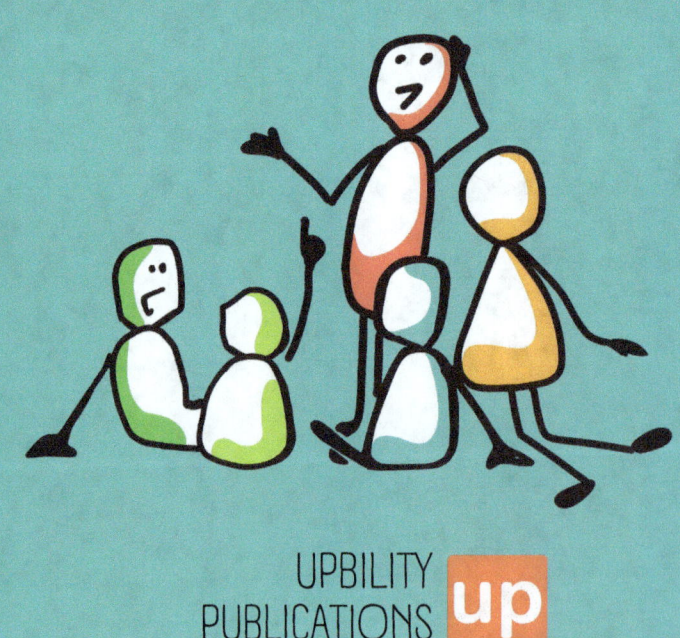

UPBILITY
PUBLICATIONS up

www.ingramcontent.com/pod-product-compliance
Lightning Source LLC
Chambersburg PA
CBHW081428220526
45466CB00008B/2305